ELEVENTH EDITION

DIABETES MELLITUS

A Practical Handbook

Sue K. Milchovich, RN, BSN, CDE

Barbara Dunn-Long, RD

T0159615

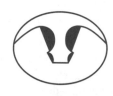

Bull Publishing
Boulder, Colorado

The use of brand names is for identifying a product and does not mean the authors recommend or promote these products.

The concept of using IDEAS (IDEAS—Understanding Your Blood Sugar, page 25) to represent insulin, diet, emotions, activity, and sickness is credited to Sally Myres, R.N., M.S. from the article, "Diabetes Management by the Patient and the Nurse Practitioner," *Nursing Clinics of North America*, Vol. 12, No. 3, September 1977.

Bull Publishing Company
P.O. Box 1377
Boulder, Colorado 80306
(800) 676-2855
www.bullpub.com

Publisher: James Bull
Cover Design: Shannon Bodie, Lightbourne Images

Library of Congress Cataloging-in-Publication Data

Milchovich, Sue K.
    Diabetes mellitus : a practical handbook / Sue K. Milchovich, Barbara
    Dunn-Long. Eleventh edition.
        pages cm
Summary: "From proper dieting to the latest medical treatments—a complete guide to managing life with diabetes. Now updated to include the latest developments in medicine and practices for diabetes treatment, as well as the most current information on new medication delivery methods, this comprehensive guide covers every aspect of living with diabetes. This user-friendly book takes a look at both the medical and nutritional sides of the disease and teaches diabetics how to balance diet, medication, and exercise for optimal health from the start. The diet and exercise plans that are included feature portion sizes and sample meal plans along with low-impact workout routines and have been revised to reflect new food pyramid guidelines and current minimum exercise suggestions. While an absolute cure for diabetes has not yet been discovered, this health manual makes living with the disease manageable"—Provided by publisher.
ISBN 978-1-936693-86-3 (paperback)
1. Diabetes—Handbooks, manuals, etc. I. Dunn-Long, Barbara. II. Title.
    RC660.5.M54 2015
    616.4'62—dc23
                                                            2015022597
Printed in the United States.

Eleventh edition

19 18 17 16 15   10 9 8 7 6 5 4 3 2 1

Contents

Acknowledgments   vi
Preface   vii
About the Authors   viii
Survival Skills   ix
The Circle of Good Diabetes Control   x

CHAPTER 1
Diabetes Mellitus   1
  Heredity 2 ■ *Viruses and the Immune System* 2 ■ *Nutrition and Obesity* 3 ■ *Types of Diabetes* 4 ■ *Glucose and Insulin* 7

CHAPTER 2
Hyperglycemia   13

CHAPTER 3
Hypoglycemia   15
  Glucagon Injection 21 ■ *Please Read This Story* 22

CHAPTER 4
IDEAS—Understanding Your Blood Sugar   25
  Acceptable or Target Blood Sugar Range 28

CHAPTER 5
Diet   29
  Type 1 Diabetes 31 ■ *Type 2 Diabetes and Overweight* 31
  Timing 32 ■ *Amounts of Foods/Calories* 33 ■ *What Is a Healthy Weight?* 34 ■ *Meal Planning* 37 ■ *Exchange Lists for Meal Planning* 42 ■ *Sample Meal Plans* 77 ■ *Alternative Sweeteners* 82 ■ *Understanding Food Labels* 84 ■ *Alcohol* 88
  Shopping Tips 89 ■ *Dining Out in Restaurants* 90 ■ *Saturated Fat and Cholesterol* 99 ■ *Fiber in Your Diet* 102 ■ *Meal Planning Resources* 107

CHAPTER 6
Home Blood Sugar Testing   111

CHAPTER 7
Ketones and Keto-Acidosis   119

CHAPTER 8
Medicines to Treat Diabetes   123
  Oral Medicines 124 ■ Insulin 134
  The Insulin Syringe 139 ■ Injection Technique 140

CHAPTER 9
Laboratory Tests   149
  Fasting Blood Sugar 149 ■ Post-Prandial Blood Sugar 149
  Estimated Average Glucose (eAG) 150

CHAPTER 10
Exercise   153
  The Benefits 153 ■ The Types 154 ■ The Parts of an Exercise
  Program 155 ■ How Hard to Exercise 156 ■ How Often to
  Exercise 160 ■ When to Exercise 160 ■ When Not to
  Exercise 161 ■ Warning Signs to Stop Exercise 161
  Guidelines for Exercising 162 ■ Sources of Information on
  Exercise 163

CHAPTER 11
Sick Days   165

CHAPTER 12
Personal Hygiene   169
  Skin Care 170 ■ Foot Care 171

CHAPTER 13
Medical Identification   173

CHAPTER 14
Stress   175

CHAPTER 15
Emotions—They Are a Part of Us   *179*

CHAPTER 16
Traveling with Diabetes   *183*
  Sources of Additional Helpful Information   185

CHAPTER 17
Complications of Diabetes   *187*
  Heart and Blood Vessel Disease   188   ▪   Nerves   188
  Eyes   189   ▪   Kidneys   191   ▪   Teeth and Gums   192
  Smoking   192

CHAPTER 18
Research on Diabetes   *195*

CHAPTER 19
Organizations and Resources   *199*
  Web Page Addresses   201   ▪   Apps for Diabetes   202
  dLife TV   197   ▪   Books   197

APPENDIX A
Answers to Quiz on Hyperglycemia and Hypoglycemia   *207*

APPENDIX B
Meal Planning Forms   *209*

APPENDIX C
Bibliography   *213*

Index   *217*

Acknowledgments

We especially wish to recognize and express our appreciation to Herbert I. Rettinger, M.D., editor for the early editions of this book; to Saundra J. Emerson, R.N., for her contributions to the original writing of this book, and to Andrea D. Manes, Charlotte L. Penington, Beverly Worcester, R.N., Beatrice Edquist, R.N., and Susan Magrann, M.S., R.D., for their valuable contributions.

S.K.M. and B.D.L.

Sometimes it is so difficult to put thoughts into words, but at this time I wish to express my deepest and most sincere thanks to my husband, Dan, and my friend, Sue Bermond-Perry. If it had not been for their constant encouragement and understanding and critical review of the manuscript, I probably would have given up long ago on this project. I thank you from the bottom of my heart.

—Sue

Preface

Diabetes. Do you recall your immediate reaction to that word when someone said it to you for the first time? Most likely you were shocked or depressed. Perhaps you even denied that such a thing could happen to you. "Why me?" was probably something that you kept repeating to yourself until reality began to sink in. From that moment on you may have realized countless, sometimes drastic changes in your lifestyle. Having diabetes is not easy. Neither is coping with it if lack of knowledge and fear are your only tools.

DIABETES MELLITUS: A Practical Handbook is *must* reading. It explains diabetes in simple language and diagrams. With proper understanding diabetes becomes easier to live with and control. The knowledge and guidelines presented in this book are essential for all those who want to help themselves or someone they know and love.

S.K.M. and B.D.L.

About the Authors

Suellyn K. Milchovich, RN, BSN, CDE, is a Certified Diabetes Nurse Educator for HealthCare Partners Medical Group, a member of the American Diabetes Association, and a member of the American Association of Diabetes Educators.

Barbara Dunn-Long, RD, is in private practice and is a member of the American Diabetes Association as well as the American Dietetic Association.

Survival Skills

See pages 205–206 for resource centers where you can
purchase the books mentioned throughout this book.

THE CIRCLE OF GOOD DIABETES CONTROL

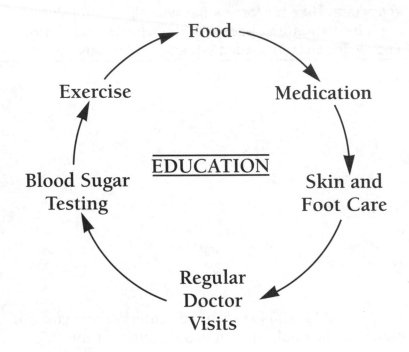

Diabetes Mellitus

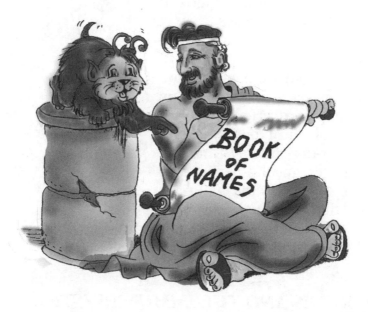

Diabetes mellitus has been known to man since about 2000–3000 B.C. The Greeks and Romans gave diabetes its name:

DIABETES = SIPHON (frequent urination)

MELLITUS = HONEY (sugar in the urine)

At the present time, diabetes affects about 21 million Americans. As long as more and more people become over-weight, and as we live longer, we will continue to see an increase in the number of people with diabetes. It is esti-mated that for every person who is *known* to have diabetes there is one person who does not know.

HEREDITY

Diabetes is not a contagious disease. You cannot catch it from or give it to anyone. Heredity plays a very important role in its occurrence. It is believed that the susceptibility to diabetes is passed from generation to generation via genes, but not in any specific pattern. Heredity plays a stronger role in Type 2 diabetes (non-insulin-dependent) than in Type 1 diabetes (insulin-dependent) (see pages 4–5), but the nature of these genetic factors and how they 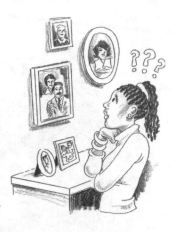 are inherited are not yet understood. You may or may not know of other family members who have diabetes.

VIRUSES AND THE IMMUNE SYSTEM

Understanding the way the human body's immune system works may someday answer a lot of questions about the cause of Type 1 diabetes (insulin-dependent). The immune system normally works to protect the body from harmful viruses and bacteria, but, for reasons not completely under-stood, in some people this protective system fails. It begins to destroy the cells of the pancreas that make insulin, so the body can no longer produce its own insulin.

There is also a seasonal factor in Type 1 diabetes—a greater number of people are diagnosed with it during the flu and virus season.

NUTRITION AND OBESITY

There is a direct connection between being overweight and having Type 2 diabetes (non-insulin-dependent). The pancreas of a person with Type 2 diabetes produces insulin, but the excess weight prevents the body cells or tissues from using it. We call this INSULIN RESISTANCE. Many times a person will also have high blood pressure and high cholesterols forming what is called the "Insulin Resistance Syndrome." Losing weight and exercising can result in the body's cells or tissues once again being able to use the insulin made by the pancreas. Blood sugars, blood pressure, and cholesterol all drop to healthier levels.

Currently there is a rapid rise in the number of people in the world with Type 2 diabetes, including teenagers and children. This type of diabetes occurs more often in people who:

- Have family members with diabetes
- Are overweight
- Have high blood pressure
- Have high cholesterols, especially high triglycerides and low HDL (see page 193)
- Are Hispanic American
- Are African American
- Are Native American
- Are Asian/Pacific Islander American
- Have had diabetes during pregnancy (gestational diabetes)
- Have had large babies (over nine pounds)

These are called the *risk factors* for diabetes. How many do you have? How many do your family members have?

TYPES OF DIABETES

Type 1 Diabetes (Insulin-Dependent)

- Formerly called juvenile diabetes
- Usually occurs before age 20 but can occur at any age
- Affects 10% of the total diabetes population
- No insulin production in the pancreas
- Has some connection to heredity
- Affects males and females equally
- Rapid weight loss
- Many symptoms plus ketones
- Seasonal: more often diagnosed during flu season
- Treatment:

  Insulin: learning how to adjust insulin for changes in eating, exercise, illness, or pregnancy

  Personal plan of meals and snacks to allow "usual" or ethnic foods

  Good nutrition meeting needs for growth or pregnancy (and breastfeeding)

  Exercise

  Education

Type 2 Diabetes (Non-Insulin-Dependent)

- Formerly called maturity onset diabetes
- Occurs in adults and children
- Affects 90% of the total diabetes population
- Insulin is made by pancreas, but there is not enough or the body cannot use it correctly
- Has strong connection to heredity and being overweight
- Is slow to develop
- Majority are overweight, few are normal weight
- Has no seasonal connection
- Treatment: Weight loss (if overweight)

    Maintain weight (if weight is good)

    Personal plan of meals and/or snacks to:

    - Include "usual" or ethnic foods
    - Adjusted for work, school, activities
    - Work for target blood sugars
    - Work for normal levels of blood fats (cholesterol and triglycerides)
    - Work for normal blood pressure

    Exercise

    Oral medication and/or insulin if needed

    Education

At Risk for Diabetes

- Also known as Impaired Fasting Glucose or Impaired Glucose Tolerance
- Formerly called borderline diabetes
- Have fasting blood sugars over 100 but under 126 mg/dl
- In a glucose tolerance test, have a 2 hour blood sugar between 140–199 mg/dl
- Have a Hemoglobin A1c result 5.7%–6.4%
- Are usually overweight
- Have insulin resistance
- Treatment: Healthy eating for weight loss
            Normal blood sugars
            Normal blood fats (cholesterol and triglycerides)
            Normal blood pressure
        Exercise
        Education

Gestational Diabetes

- Occurs during pregnancy, in the last trimester
- Have insulin resistance
- Many pregnant women are tested between 24 and 28 weeks of pregnancy
- Treatment: diet and sometimes insulin
- Good control of blood sugars is an absolute must to protect the baby
- Blood sugars usually return to normal once the baby is born.
- Many women develop diabetes later
- It is important to maintain normal weight

GLUCOSE AND INSULIN

In order to control your blood sugar, you must understand *glucose* and *insulin*.

- Glucose, or sugar → comes from the food you eat
  raises blood sugar
- Insulin → is made by the pancreas
  helps the liver, muscle, and fat cells use glucose
  must have enough of it and it must be working correctly

Let's Start with GLUCOSE

All the foods we eat consist of CARBOHYDRATES, PROTEINS, and FATS.

- CARBOHYDRATES (see pages 43–55) include:
  Foods high in sugar—"sweets," honey, syrup, sugar, etc.
  Starches—cereals, bread, potatoes, rice, pasta, corn, peas, beans, etc.
  Fruits
  Milk, yogurt

- PROTEINS (see pages 57–63) include:
  Meat—poultry, beef, fish, etc.
  Eggs
  Cheese, cottage cheese
  Peanut butter
  Tofu

■ **FATS** (see pages 63–65) include:

Oils

Margarine and butter

Salad dressing

Mayonnaise

Bacon

Avocado

Nuts and seeds

The stomach and intestines break down 100% of all the CARBOHYDRATES you eat to glucose. This glucose enters the blood, causing your blood sugar to rise. Be aware of the TOTAL AMOUNT of carbohydrate foods you eat at any one time.

Eat a large amount of carbohydrate foods. → Blood sugar rises too high.

Eat little or no carbohydrate foods. → Blood sugar may drop too low.

Your blood sugar will remain more stable if you keep the TOTAL AMOUNT of carbohydrate foods eaten from meal to meal constant and balance them with some protein, fat, and vegetables. Do not focus on the sugar content of foods—look at the TOTAL CARBOHYDRATE amount (see nutrition label on page 87).

Vegetables contain carbohydrates, but because they have so few calories and little carbohydrate, they do not affect blood sugar unless eaten in large amounts.

PROTEIN does not affect blood sugar. The type and amount of protein foods you choose to eat depend on what you need to do about your weight (lose, gain, or maintain) and whether your cholesterol is high or normal.

INCLUDE A SMALL AMOUNT OF PROTEIN WITH EACH MEAL to help control the rise in blood sugar that occurs after eating and help you go 4 to 5 hours between meals.

FAT does not cause blood sugar to rise. The type and amount of fat you choose to eat depend on what you need to do about your weight (lose, gain, or maintain) and whether your cholesterol is high or normal. A meal that is high in fat (for example, pizza) will keep your blood sugar *up longer*.

The "perfect meal" is made up of *small amounts* of foods from *all the groups*.

AMOUNT IS THE KEY![1]

Insulin

INSULIN is a hormone made in the pancreas, which is located behind and below the stomach.

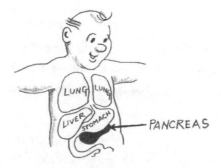

When the blood sugar rises, insulin is released into the blood. Both insulin and glucose travel all over the body via the blood.

---

[1]This is the first "Survival Skills" passage. They will be shaded like this throughout the book.

In the MUSCLES, glucose is turned into ENERGY.

The LIVER stores glucose for future use (especially if blood sugar drops too low).

FAT cells take and store all the excess glucose as fat.

For glucose to enter a cell and do its work, INSULIN must be present to act as a transporter. Think of it as glucose coming upon a locked door, and insulin as the key that opens the door.

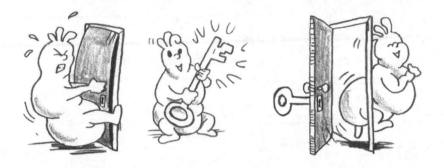

When you have diabetes, there is a problem with insulin:

■ Type 1 diabetes ➔ No insulin is produced.

The cells in the pancreas that make insulin have been destroyed by the body, so no insulin is made.

■ Type 2 diabetes ➔ Too little insulin is produced

and/or

insulin is made, but it does not work very well

Type 2 diabetes

In someone who is thin or of normal weight, the cells of the pancreas do not make enough insulin.

In those who are overweight, a lot of insulin is made at first but will decrease over time. Also the insulin does not work correctly. It cannot get into the muscle and fat cells to do its work. This is called *insulin resistance.*

There are 2 ways to break the insulin resistance and get the body to use the insulin:

- LOSE WEIGHT: 10 to 20 pounds is the "key" amount.
- EXERCISE: See exercise on pages 153–164.

Presently, the exact cause of diabetes (Type 1 and Type 2) is unknown, and there is no cure. Once you have diabetes, you have it for the rest of your life.

You will learn how to keep your blood sugars as close to normal as possible by balancing food, body weight, medication, and exercise. The best way to do this is to work with several people (no one person can teach you all you need to know) known as your "diabetes team."

You must be the center of the team. The other members may include any or all of the following people:

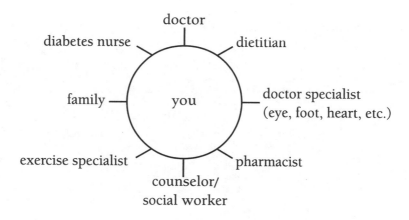

With good planning and habits, you will be able to feel your best *and* be in control of the diabetes, rather than having the diabetes control you.

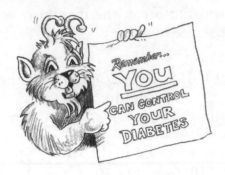

CHAPTER 2

Hyperglycemia

One problem you may have if your food, medication, and activity balance is disturbed is too much sugar in the blood. This is called **HYPERGLYCEMIA**.

HYPER = too much
GLYC = sugar   } *HYPERGLYCEMIA*
EMIA = blood

HYPERGLYCEMIA can occur

- If you forget or reduce your insulin or oral medication
- If you eat too much, especially carbohydrate foods and meals high in fat
- If you have a fever, cold, flu, infection, surgery, or other illness or emotional stress
- From "bad" medication—medication that is out of date or no longer working, or insulin that has been frozen or stored at too high a temperature
- From inactivity

The classic symptoms of hyperglycemia are

- Unusual thirst
- Frequent urination
- Fatigue, extreme tiredness
- Persistent infections

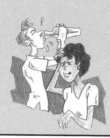

Hyperglycemia occurs slowly, and your blood sugar can rise to a fairly high level (about 300 mg/dl) before you feel these symptoms. Keep track of your blood sugars through blood and urine sugar tests.

For those of you with Type 1 diabetes, as your blood sugar rises you may also form ketones, which show up in your blood and urine (explanations of ketones, acidosis, and diabetic coma are on pages 119–121).

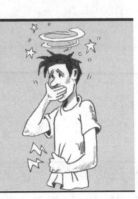

When the ketones form you begin to feel symptoms such as

- Weight loss

- Nausea and vomiting

- Abdominal cramps

- Deep, rapid breathing

- "Fruity" breath

Other names you might hear for hyperglycemia or high blood sugar are DIABETIC KETO-ACIDOSIS and DIABETIC COMA.

CHAPTER 3

Hypoglycemia

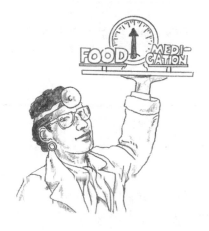

Your food, medication, and exercise must be balanced to keep the amount of sugar in your blood as close to normal as possible. If the balance is not maintained, you may have either too much or too little sugar, which could lead to serious trouble.

HYPOGLYCEMIA, INSULIN REACTION, and INSULIN SHOCK are all names for too little sugar in the bloodstream. This occurs when the blood sugar drops below 70 mg/dl or drops rapidly from a higher level to a lower level. (How to measure blood sugars is explained on pages 111–118).

HYPO = too little
GLYC = sugar   } *HYPOGLYCEMIA*
EMIA = blood

HYPOGLYCEMIA can occur

- If you take too much or are on too much insulin or oral medication
- If you eat too little or skip or delay meals and snacks
- From excessive or unplanned exercise or the timing of exercise

Hypoglycemia can occur at night while you are sleeping, especially if you take insulin. You may actually sleep through it and not awaken.

Clues to nighttime hypoglycemia are

- Bed clothes and sheets wet from sweat
- Headache on awakening
- Nightmares, restless sleeping
- Extreme fatigue on awakening
- High (fasting) blood sugars in the morning

Hypoglycemia can occur in people taking insulin or oral medications. Those who control their diabetes by diet alone usually do not develop hypoglycemia.

When you have an insulin reaction or become hypoglycemic, the symptoms will come on SUDDENLY. Some of the first symptoms are

- Cold sweats, clammy feeling
- Shakiness, dizziness, or weakness
- Irritability, crankiness, or impatience
- Heart pounding or beating faster

- Nervousness
- Hunger

When the brain senses that your blood sugar is low you may also feel

- Headache
- Numbness or tingling in the fingertips or lips
- Blurred or double vision
- Confused thinking
- Slurred speech
- Personality change
- Seizure
- Unconsciousness

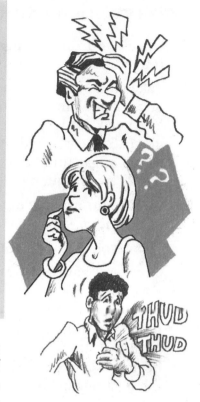

If you are hypoglycemic, you usually will have 2, 3, or 4 of these symptoms. Any one alone probably will not mean low blood sugar. If possible, test your blood sugar immediately, as soon as you feel any of the symptoms, and see if your sugar is indeed low. Regardless of how severe or numerous they may be,

TAKE HEED OF THE EARLY WARNING SYMPTOMS,

and do not wait to see if they will go away. Call your doctor when you are having repeated or severe hypoglycemic reactions.

When you experience low blood sugar, do the following:

1. Check your blood sugar immediately.

2. Take some kind of "Fast Sugar Food" immediately. You need 10–15 grams of glucose or carbohydrate to put sugar into your bloodstream quickly.

3. Limit your activity at once. Lie or sit down.

4. If possible, tell someone.

5. Once you have eaten the Fast Sugar Food, the symptoms should begin to fade (within 10 or 15 minutes). If you do not begin to feel better, repeat the Fast Sugar Food.

6. Once you are feeling normal again, it is wise to follow up with a snack, especially if more than ½ hour will pass before the next meal. If it is close to meal time, ½ hour or so, just go ahead and have your regular meal.

Example of Snack*

1 meat (see pages 57–63) or protein		1 oz. meat		2 Tbsp peanut butter
+	=	+	OR	+
1 starch (see pages 43–47)		1 slice bread		5–6 soda crackers

---

* If you have no need to lose weight, you may need to increase the amount suggested.

Examples of Fast Sugar Foods containing 10–15 grams of glucose or carbohydrate include

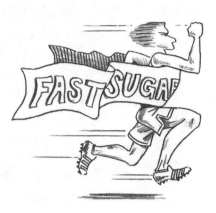

5–7 Lifesavers

4–6 ounces of orange juice or apple juice

2 ounces of grape juice

4–6 ounces of regular soda (*not diet*)

6 jelly beans

10 gumdrops

2 lumps (or teaspoons) of sugar

2 level teaspoons of honey or maple syrup

8 ounces of fat-free milk

There are also several glucose tablets and gels you can use:

Cake-decorating gel
available in grocery stores
1 tube = 10 grams glucose

Insta Glucose
available in pharmacies
1 tube = 30 grams glucose

Glutose
available in pharmacies
1 tube = 15 grams of glucose
1 multidose tube = 45 grams of glucose

Glucose tablets
available in pharmacies
1 tablet = 4 grams glucose
10 tablets/tube

GlucoBurst Gel   available in pharmacies
                        1 pouch = 15 grams of glucose
                        3 pouches/box

Dex Glucose   available in pharmacies
Gel   1 tube = 17 grams of glucose
                        3 tubes/package

Liquid Shot   available in pharmacies
                        1 bottle = 15 grams of glucose

Glucose Rapid   available in pharmacies
Spray   5–10 sprays
                        100 sprays/bottle

Quick Sticks   available in pharmacies
                        1 package = 10 grams of glucose

Level Life gel   available in pharmacies
                        1 pack = 15 grams glucose

ALWAYS carry a FAST SUGAR FOOD with you!
WHAT WILL YOU CARRY FOR YOUR FAST SUGAR
FOOD?

_____

WHERE WILL YOU CARRY IT?

_____

WHAT WILL YOU CARRY FOR A SNACK?

GLUCAGON INJECTION

GLUCAGON is a hormone that, when injected under the skin or in a muscle, raises the blood sugar level quickly. If you are found unconscious by one of your family members or friends, and you are unable to take sugar by mouth because of the danger of choking, the person caring for you can give an injection of glucagon into a muscle or in an area you would give an insulin injection (page 145). After receiving an injection of glucagon you should respond within 5 to 15 minutes. When you do respond, it is necessary to eat—bread and meat or milk—because the effects of glucagon last only an hour or so. If you have Type 1 diabetes, you may need to keep glucagon at home or carry it with you when traveling. Check the expiration date on your bottle and replace it when necessary. If glucagon is used to treat a hypoglycemic reaction, this should be reported to your doctor as soon as possible.

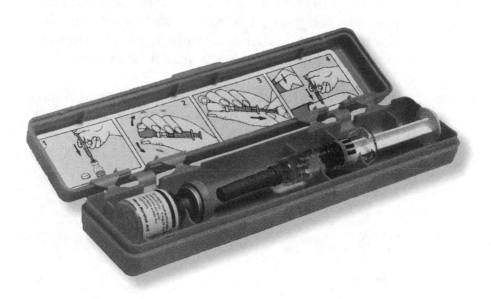

PLEASE READ THIS STORY

Just as he would any other morning, Jake Sumner took his usual dose of insulin, ate his normal breakfast, and drove to work. Jake Sumner is a high school math teacher. Because of a mandatory teachers' meeting, Jake did not have enough time to eat all of his lunch and left about half of it. That afternoon after school, several of Jake's friends decided to play nine holes of golf, and Jake joined them. At about the fourth hole, Jake felt himself becoming very irritated with the game and his fellow players. A few minutes later he became shaky and nervous and broke out in a cold sweat. Immediately his thoughts flashed back to his half-eaten lunch, his usual dose of insulin, and the extra exercise he was getting. "Insulin reaction," he thought as he searched his pockets for the Lifesavers he normally carried. No Lifesavers! Furthermore, none of his friends had any Fast Sugar Foods with them. So Jake sent one of the men to the pro shop for Lifesavers while another friend stayed with him. Luckily, the pro shop was very close and did have some Fast Sugar Food. Jake ate it quickly and within ten minutes felt much better. Instead of continuing to play, he excused himself and left for home. Jake knew that if he continued to exercise he would have another reaction. Also, to prevent another insulin reaction, Jake ate a snack of cheese and crackers, because he would not be able to eat dinner for another hour. Because of this reaction, Jake Sumner was reminded of four very important aspects of diabetes:

- You must eat your entire food allowance for each meal.
- You must carry some form of Fast Sugar Food with you at all times.
- Exercise helps make the insulin you are taking work more effectively, allowing glucose into the cells.
- If you cannot eat a meal within the next 30 minutes, you must eat a snack that includes a serving from the bread and meat groups.

Q U I Z
Hyperglycemia and Hypoglycemia

Here is a quiz on hyperglycemia and hypoglycemia. See if you can answer the questions without looking at your notes. The answers are listed on page 207).

1. Write in HYPER or HYPO or BOTH in the space next to each item.
   a. Drowsiness or listlessness _____
   b. Happens suddenly _____
   c. Headache _____
   d. Thirst _____
   e. Nausea, vomiting _____
   f. Infection _____
   g. Deep, rapid breathing _____
   h. Too little food _____
   i. Forgotten insulin _____
   j. Fever, cold _____
   k. Impatient, irritable _____
   l. Overexercise _____
   m. Blurred vision _____
   n. Heart pounding _____

2. Circle the letters that are symptoms of an insulin reaction or low blood sugar.
   a. Urinating more than usual
   b. Shakiness, nervousness
   c. Irritability
   d. Abdominal cramps
   e. Sweating, clamminess
   f. Blurred vision

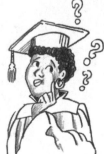

CHAPTER 4

IDEAS
Understanding Your Blood Sugar

Everything you do and everything that happens to you affects your blood sugar. Remembering the key word IDEAS will help you understand why your blood sugar is too high, too low, or acceptable (within a range of blood sugars that you and your doctor have agreed is best for you).

I stands for *Insulin* and/or oral medication

D stands for *Diet* or food

E stands for *Emotions*

A stands for *Activity* or exercise

S stands for *Sickness*

FOOD, MEDICATION, and EXERCISE can be thought of as tools to use to "balance" or control your blood sugar. Picture a seesaw:

FOOD   MEDICATION   EXERCISE

△

You want to keep these three balanced so your blood sugar stays in your acceptable range. Home blood-glucose testing will let you know if your blood sugars are indeed in that acceptable range or whether they are out of balance.

When something disturbs your food, medication, or exercise, or you become ill or suffer emotional stress, the seesaw tips and your blood sugar goes too high or too low.

The following chart will help you understand what upsets the seesaw, throwing blood sugars out of balance. The *IDEAS* are listed down the center of the page. On the left side are those events that raise the blood sugar; on the right are those that lower it. Many times you will find more than one event tipping your seesaw and upsetting your blood sugar balance.

Events Raising Blood Sugar	*Events* Lowering Blood Sugar
Insulin or Oral Medication	
Forget to take medication	Take too much medication
Not on enough medication*	On too much medication*
"Bad" medication (out of date, stored in temperatures above 80°F or frozen)	Timing

*The amount of medication your doctor has prescribed is either too much or too little for you.

Events Raising Blood Sugar	*Events* Lowering Blood Sugar
Medication no longer working	
Timing	

Diet/Food

Eat too much	Eat too little
Sugary foods (includes fruit) eaten alone	Skip meals/ snacks
Meals high in fat	Delay meals/snacks
Meals not well balanced	Meals not well balanced
Meals/snacks too close together	Meals/snacks too far apart

Emotions

Traumatic emotions, such as loss of loved one, accident, surgery, or major illness	None

Activity

Inactivity	Too much or unplanned exercise
	Exercise just before a meal
	Exercise at same time insulin is peaking

Events Raising Blood Sugar		*Events* Lowering Blood Sugar
	Sickness	
Cold, flu, fever, pain, infection, major illness, surgery, some dental work		None
IDEAS in balance	➔	blood sugars in your acceptable range.
IDEAS out of balance	➔	blood sugars too high or too low.

Keep this listing handy so you can refer to it readily when you are trying to understand your particular blood sugar levels and their pattern.

ACCEPTABLE OR TARGET BLOOD SUGAR RANGE

You should talk with your doctor or diabetes educator to decide what is the best TARGET BLOOD SUGAR RANGE for you. You may use the following as a guideline:

Fasting or before meals	80–130
2 hours after a meal or at bedtime	Less than 180
Estimated Average Glucose (eAG) (Hemoglobin A1c) (see pages 150–152)	Generally 6.5–7% but discuss with your health care provider

CHAPTER 5

Diet

DIET IS THE CORNERSTONE OF BLOOD SUGAR CONTROL.

Having diabetes does not mean that you must give up all the foods you like, but it does mean that you must pay more attention to the types of food you eat and when you eat.

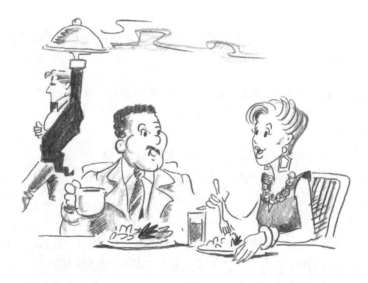

In most cases you will be given a meal plan to follow to help keep your blood sugar in balance. The type of diabetes you have (Type 1 or Type 2) helps determine this meal plan. Do not think of the meal plan as a diet but rather as a GUIDE TO HEALTHY EATING!

Dietary Guidelines for Americans (written by the U.S. Departments of Agriculture and Health and Human Services) recommends basic good nutrition for EVERYONE for the purpose of improving health and preventing long-term diseases (such as heart disease, high blood pressure, and some cancers).

When you have diabetes, following these guidelines is an important first step in lowering your blood sugar and learning how to make HEALTHY FOOD CHOICES. The biggest advantage is that your whole family can eat healthier along with you. **Making healthy food choices** can ensure that you will be able to:

- Keep your weight normal
- Keep your blood glucose normal
- Keep your blood fat levels normal

When you are planning your meals, it will help your diabetes if you:

- Eat the right amount of food at the right times, and don't skip meals. Keep the amount of carbohydrate foods constant from meal to meal.
- Eat a variety of foods and make HEALTHY FOOD CHOICES. Include plenty of whole-grain products, vegetables, and fruits and a moderate amount of protein.
- Substitute nonfat dairy products for high-fat ones.
- Eat less fat, especially saturated fat, and cholesterol (see page 101). This will help keep your blood fat levels down.
- Avoid Trans fatty acids (trans fats).
- Use less sugar. Limit special treats, candies, and sweet desserts. These foods provide no nutritional value, have added fat, and few vitamins and minerals.

TYPE 1 DIABETES

If you have Type 1 diabetes, you need to work with your dietitian to create a meal plan that allows you to make adjustments in your diet during exercise, illness, and pregnancy and on special occasions. Teenagers with Type 1 diabetes need to have meals planned so that their special growth needs are met.

You should also work very closely with your doctor and diabetes nurse educator to learn how your insulin works. Once you understand this, you can learn how to make adjustments in your insulin to handle changes in blood sugar during exercise, eating changes, special occasions, illness, pregnancy, and the growth periods of teens.

Knowing how to make these adjustments in your insulin and food allows you to keep better control of your blood sugar. Remember:

- Keep your weight constant. If you are a child or teenager, your weight should be in a good range for your age.
- Good nutrition leads to good health.
- Stick to your personal plan for meals and snacks, which is matched with the time and action of your insulin.

TYPE 2 DIABETES AND OVERWEIGHT

If you have Type 2 diabetes and are overweight, it is very important for you to lose weight and keep it off! You do not have to get down to your ideal body weight, but losing as much as 10 to 20 pounds will lower your blood sugar. Many people who have diabetes also have high blood pressure and high blood fat (cholesterol and triglyceride) levels. Weight loss will not only lower your blood sugar but will also work to lower your blood pressure and blood fat levels.

To help yourself lose weight and eat healthy:

- Lower the total amount of fat you eat.
- Eat smaller portions.
- Eat reduced-fat and low-calorie snacks (check labels).
- Increase the fiber in your diet.
- Be more active. Get out and enjoy life—take a walk, go for a swim, dance, whatever you enjoy.

If you have high blood pressure, you will be asked to eat foods low in sodium (salt).

TIMING

The TIMING of your meals and snacks is important to balance the food you eat with the medication you are taking. Try to eat your meals and snacks at about the same time every day. Do not skip meals or save portions from one meal for a later meal. Try to eat about the same amount of food from day to day.

Example

Breakfast	7:00–9:00 A.M.	
Lunch	11:30 A.M.–1:30 P.M.	
Supper	5:00–7:00 P.M.	
Snack	9:30–10:30 P.M.	

AMOUNTS OF FOODS/CALORIES

The AMOUNTS of different foods you eat will depend on your AGE, WEIGHT, and ACTIVITY. All adults need to consume the right number of calories to keep their weight normal and their diabetes under control. This includes additional calories during pregnancy and while breastfeeding. Children and teenagers need to consume the right amount of calories for normal growth and development.

Your doctor or dietitian will determine the number of calories you need each day. The dietitian translates these CALORIES into your very own meal plan, which is usually divided into three meals and as many snacks as you need. It will tell you the number of servings you need from each exchange or choice list for each meal and snack.

Measuring Foods

At first you should measure all foods to be sure of the amounts. Use a standard 8-ounce measuring cup, measuring teaspoon, and a measuring tablespoon. Most foods are measured after cooking. Later as you become more familiar with your meal plan, you will be able to estimate portion sizes without having to measure. Even so, our eyes cannot always be trusted, and the portion sizes you are judging by eye may grow larger or smaller as time passes. To check yourself, try to measure your portion sizes every six months.

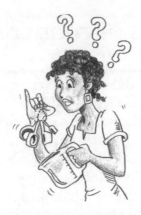

Common Measurement Equivalents

   3 tsp. = 1 Tbsp.

   4 Tbsp. = ¼ cup

   5 ½ Tbsp. = ⅓ cup

   4 ounces = ½ cup

   8 ounces = 1 cup

Nutrition labels and diet cookbooks measure ingredients in grams. A simple way to understand this is that 28.4 grams equal 1 ounce of food. For example, if 100 grams is listed, that is equal to about 4 ounces.

WHAT IS A HEALTHY WEIGHT?

Your doctor or dietitian may use a useful tool called the BMI (body mass index) to determine if you are at a healthy weight. Having too much body fat can cause insulin resistance. Losing weight and increasing the amount of muscle you have while decreasing the amount of body fat helps your body use insulin better.

Body Mass Index Table

BMI	Normal							Overweight				Obese										Extreme Obesity														
Height (Inches)	19	20	21	22	23	24	25	26	27	28	29	30	31	32	33	34	35	36	37	38	39	40	41	42	43	44	45	46	47	48	49	50	51	52	53	54
												Body Weight (pounds)																									
58	91	96	100	105	110	115	119	124	129	134	138	143	148	153	158	162	167	172	177	181	186	191	196	201	205	210	215	220	224	229	234	239	244	248	253	258
59	94	99	104	109	114	119	124	128	133	138	143	148	153	158	163	168	173	178	183	188	193	198	203	208	212	217	222	227	232	237	242	247	252	257	262	267
60	97	102	107	112	118	123	128	133	138	143	148	153	158	163	168	174	179	184	189	194	199	204	209	215	220	225	230	235	240	245	250	255	261	266	271	276
61	100	106	111	116	122	127	132	137	143	148	153	158	164	169	174	180	185	190	195	201	206	211	217	222	227	232	238	243	248	254	259	264	269	275	280	285
62	104	109	115	120	126	131	136	142	147	153	158	164	169	175	180	186	191	196	202	207	213	218	224	229	235	240	246	251	256	262	267	273	278	284	289	295
63	107	113	118	124	130	135	141	146	152	158	163	169	175	180	186	191	197	203	208	214	220	225	231	237	242	248	254	259	265	270	278	282	287	293	299	304
64	110	116	122	128	134	140	145	151	157	163	169	174	180	186	192	197	204	209	215	221	227	232	238	244	250	256	262	267	273	279	285	291	296	302	308	314
65	114	120	126	132	138	144	150	156	162	168	174	180	186	192	198	204	210	216	222	228	234	240	246	252	258	264	270	276	282	288	294	300	306	312	318	324
66	118	124	130	136	142	148	155	161	167	173	179	186	192	198	204	210	216	223	229	235	241	247	253	260	266	272	278	284	291	297	303	309	315	322	328	334
67	121	127	134	140	146	153	159	166	172	178	185	191	198	204	211	217	223	230	236	242	249	255	261	268	274	280	287	293	299	306	312	319	325	331	338	344
68	125	131	138	144	151	158	164	171	177	184	190	197	203	210	216	223	230	236	243	249	256	262	269	276	282	289	295	302	308	315	322	328	335	341	348	354
69	128	135	142	149	155	162	169	176	182	189	196	203	209	216	223	230	236	243	250	257	263	270	277	284	291	297	304	311	318	324	331	338	345	351	358	365
70	132	139	146	153	160	167	174	181	188	195	202	209	216	222	229	236	243	250	257	264	271	278	285	292	299	306	313	320	327	334	341	348	355	362	369	376
71	136	143	150	157	165	172	179	186	193	200	208	215	222	229	236	243	250	257	265	272	279	286	293	301	308	315	322	329	338	343	351	358	365	372	379	386
72	140	147	154	162	169	177	184	191	199	206	213	221	228	235	242	250	258	265	272	279	287	294	302	309	316	324	331	338	346	353	361	368	375	383	390	397
73	144	151	159	166	174	182	189	197	204	212	219	227	235	242	250	257	265	272	280	288	295	302	310	318	325	333	340	348	355	363	371	378	386	393	401	408
74	148	155	163	171	179	186	194	202	210	218	225	233	241	249	256	264	272	280	287	295	303	311	319	326	334	342	350	358	365	373	381	389	396	404	412	420
75	152	160	168	176	184	192	200	208	216	224	232	240	248	256	264	272	279	287	295	303	311	319	327	335	343	351	359	367	375	383	391	399	407	415	423	431
76	156	164	172	180	189	197	205	213	221	230	238	246	254	263	271	279	287	295	304	312	320	328	336	344	353	361	369	377	385	394	402	410	418	426	435	443

Source: Adapted from Clinical Guidelines on the Identification, Evaluation, and Treatment of Overweight and Obesity in Adults: The Evidence Report.

How to Determine Your Body Mass Index (BMI)

BMI measures your weight and how it compares to your height.

Your BMI should fall within the healthy range of 19 to 25.

If you are at the upper end of this range or more than 25, your doctor or dietitian may suggest losing enough weight to lower your BMI one or two numbers. A BMI of more than 26 is considered overweight. A BMI of 30 is considered obese. Research shows that as your BMI levels go up, blood pressure and total cholesterol levels increase, and HDL or good cholesterol levels decrease.

How BMI Is Calculated

1. Multiply your weight in pounds by 704.
   (Example: 704 × 123 pounds = 86,592)
   Your answer: _____

2. Multiply your height in inches by your height in inches.
   (Example: 60 inches × 60 inches = 3,600)
   Your answer: _____

3. To get your BMI, divide your answer in step 1 by your answer in step 2.
   (Example: 86,592 ÷ 3,600 = 24)
   Your BMI: _____

MEAL PLANNING

The three groups of foods you must think about are:

CARBOHYDRATES
PROTEINS
FATS

We will explain each of these in detail.

Carbohydrates

Carbohydrate is your body's main energy source, it keeps your heart beating, and it gives you the energy to walk up stairs. It is an important part of a healthy eating plan and affects your blood glucose levels more than any other food. The starch and sugar in the foods you eat are carbohydrates. Starch is found in breads, pasta, cereals, potatoes, peas, beans, and lentils. Naturally present sugars are in fruits, milk, and some vegetables. Added sugars are found in desserts, candy, jams, and syrups. Studies have shown that the total number of grams of carbohydrate in a meal is more important than whether some of the carbohydrates come from sugar. Sugar and foods that contain sugar must be exchanged for other carbohydrates and foods, not just added to the meal plan.

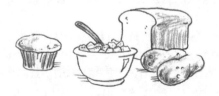 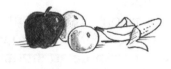

In 1995 the American Diabetes and Dietetic Associations put the old choices of bread/starch, fruit, vegetable, and milk exchanges into one group called the Carbohydrate

Group. Most of the carbohydrates we eat come from three food groups: starch, fruit, and milk. Each of the these groups contain about 15 grams of carbohydrate per serving. Milk has 12 grams of carbohydrate per serving, but you can round the carbohydrate value up to 15 to make meal planning easier. You can exchange the starch, fruit, and milk choices in your meal plan. Vegetables are in the carbohydrate group but only contain about 5 grams of carbohydrate per serving, so three servings of vegetables contain 15 grams of carbohydrate. (One or two servings of vegetables do not need to be counted.)

Each of the following is an example of 1 carbohydrate:

1 starch = 1 small potato *or* ½ cup beans

1 fruit = ½ banana *or* 1 small apple

1 milk = 1 cup milk *or* 1 cup yogurt

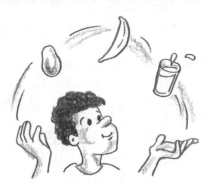

How much carbohydrate should you eat, and what is carbohydrate counting?

A healthy meal plan usually includes 3–4 carbohydrate choices at each meal and 1–2 carbohydrate choices for your snacks.

Carbohydrate counting is a way of figuring out how much carbohydrate to eat at meals and snacks. The reason you pay more attention to counting grams of carbohydrate is that carbohydrates tend to have the greatest effect on your blood sugar. As the carbohydrate is broken down into glucose and absorbed, the amount of glucose in your blood goes up. In carbohydrate counting, a serving from any of the carbohydrate groups (starches, fruit, and milk) is equal to 1 serving or 15 grams. That means that if your food plan calls for 2 starches, 1 fruit, and 1 milk at lunch, you have a total of 4 carbohydrate choices (60 grams).

2 starches + 1 fruit + 1 milk = 4 carbohydrate choices (60 grams)

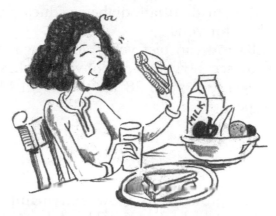

The table below shows how to count the number of grams of carbohydrate on a food label into your meal plan.

Total Carbohydrate (grams in one serving)	How to Count
0–5 grams	do not count
6–10 grams	$\frac{1}{2}$ carbohydrate choice
11–20 grams	1 carbohydrate choice
21–25 grams	$1\frac{1}{2}$ carbohydrate choices
26–35 grams	2 carbohydrate choices

Carbohydrates and Blood Glucose

The more carbohydrates you eat the more your blood glucose will go up. Some foods contain more carbohydrate than others, even though the serving size is the same.

Different type of carbohydrates vary in the time it takes your body to break them down. Cooked food is digested faster than raw. Foods mixed with liquid are digested faster than dry. Combination foods, carbohydrate mixed with fat, may take longer to digest and your blood glucose may rise slower.

Discuss with your dietitian, diabetes educator, or doctor what works best for you.

REMEMBER: You can test your blood sugar two hours after a meal to see how the carbohydrates have affected your blood sugar. See page 28 for the target blood sugar range after a meal.

Proteins

Your body uses proteins to grow and maintain tissues. Proteins are found in both vegetable and animal sources, including meat, poultry, fish, milk and other dairy products, eggs, and dried beans, peas, and nuts. Starches and vegetables also contain small amounts of protein. Your body needs insulin to use the protein you eat.

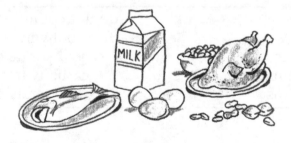

Fats

The amount of calories you should get from fat depends on your own special needs—your cholesterol level and your weight. Fats are important because they carry vitamins and important fatty acids in the body. To keep your heart and blood vessels healthy, choose fats that are polyunsaturated or monounsaturated, and avoid saturated and trans fats (see "Saturated Fat and Cholesterol," pages 99–101).

<u>Use These:</u>

Monounsaturated fats:
Avocados
Olive oil
Canola oil
Nuts: almonds, peanuts, cashews, hazelnuts, peanut butter

Polyunsaturated fats:
Corn oil
Soybean oil
Sunflower oil
Soft margarine
Safflower oil
Cottonseed oil
Flax seeds
Walnuts

Avoid These:

Saturated fat:
Coconut oil
Meat fat
Bacon
Cocoa butter (Chocolate)
Cream cheese
Hardened shortening
Sour cream
Palm oils

Trans fats:
Products containing hydro- genated oil
Processed baked goods (muffins, cookies)
Processed snack foods (crackers, chips)
Shortening
Palm oil
Fast food French fries
Solid stick margarine

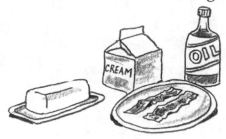

REMEMBER: All fats are high in calories. Limit serving sizes when making **healthy food choices.**

EXCHANGE LISTS FOR MEAL PLANNING

To make meal planning easier for you, carbohydrate, protein, and fat foods have been placed into food groups called the EXCHANGE or CHOICES SYSTEM. An exchange or choice is a measured amount of food selected from a group of foods. The lists provide you with a wide variety of foods to choose from. Once you become familiar with these lists, your meal planning will become easier.

There are three main groups in this system:

- Carbohydrate group, which contains
    starch
    fruit
    milk
    other carbohydrates
    vegetables
- Meat and meat substitutes group
- Fat group

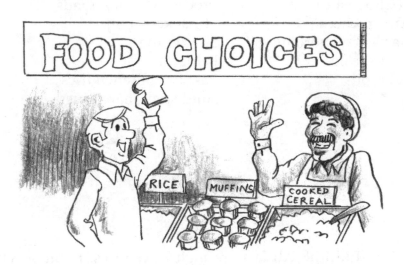

Carbohydrates

Starch choices

*In the following list, one starch choice contains 15 grams of carbohydrate, 3 grams of protein, and 80 calories. Whole-grain foods contain about 2 grams of fiber per serving (those that have 3 or more grams of fiber per serving are marked with a * symbol).*

In this list, whole-grain and enriched breads and cereals, wheat germ and bran products, and dried beans and peas are good sources of iron and among the better sources of thiamine. Whole-grain, bran, and wheat germ products have more fiber than products made from refined flours. Dried beans and peas are also good sources of fiber. Wheat germ, bran, dried beans, potatoes, lima beans, parsnips, pumpkin, and winter squash are good sources of potassium.

Starchy vegetables are included in this list because they contain the same amount of carbohydrate and protein as one slice of bread.

One starch choice is equal to any one of the following. If you wish to eat a starch food that is not on this list, the general rule for one starch choice is:

$1/2$ cup of a cereal, grain, pasta, or starchy vegetable

1 oz. of a bread food, such as 1 slice of bread

$3/4$ to 1 oz. of most snack foods (Some snack foods may have added fat, so check the label.)

Bread

bread, white, whole-wheat,
pumpernickel, rye, raisin (unfrosted) . . . . . . 1 slice (1 oz.)
bread, reduced calorie . . . . 2 slices (1½ oz.)
bagel, small (4 oz.) . . . . $1/4$ (1 oz.)
English muffin, small . . . . $1/2$ (1 oz.)

Bread (cont.)

plain roll	1 (1 oz.)
hot dog bun	$^1/_2$ (1 oz.)
hamburger bun	$^1/_2$ (1 oz.)
dried bread crumbs	2 Tbsp.
tortilla, corn or flour, 6"	1
tortilla, flour 10" across.	$^1/_3$
bread sticks (8" long, $^1/_2$" diameter)	1 stick
croutons, no fat added.	1 cup
pita, 6" across	$^1/_2$

Cereal

*bran cereals, flaked (All Bran, Bran Buds) . .	$^1/_2$ cup
other ready-to-eat, unsweetened cereals	$^3/_4$ cup
oats.	$^1/_2$ cup
Grapenuts	$^1/_4$ cup
puffed cereal (unfrosted).	$1^1/_2$ cups
cereal (cooked)	$^1/_2$ cup
grits (cooked)	$^1/_2$ cup
shredded wheat	$^1/_2$ cup
Kasha	$^1/_2$ cup
Muesli	$^1/_4$ cup

Grains/Pasta

rice, white or brown (cooked)	$^1/_3$ cup
pasta (cooked): spaghetti, noodles, macaroni	$^1/_3$ cup
cornmeal (dry).	2 Tbsp.
cornbread (2" × 2" × 1").	1 average (2 oz.)
flour.	$2^1/_2$ Tbsp.

---

*3 grams or more of fiber per serving

Grains/Pasta (cont.)

*wheat germ	3 Tbsp.
corn starch	2 Tbsp.
bulgur (cooked)	$^1/_2$ cup
couscous	$^1/_2$ cup

Crackers/Snacks

animal crackers	8
graham, $2^1/_2$" square	3
melba toast, rectangle	4 slices
matzo	$^3/_4$ oz.
oyster crackers	24
popcorn (popped, no fat added)	3 cups
pretzel sticks, $3^1/_3$" long, $^1/_8$" round	25 ($^3/_4$ oz.)
Rye Crisp, 2" × $3^1/_2$"	4
saltine crackers	6
soda cracker, $2^1/_2$" square	4

Low-Fat Crackers/Snacks—Try to use crackers that have less than 3 grams of fat per serving. Remember to check the labels!

low-fat cheese crackers, 3 grams fat	12 small
low-fat (50%) crackers, 1.5 grams fat	15 small
reduced-fat, baked wheat, 1.5 grams fat	5 wafers
whole wheat crisp breads, (such as Kavli, Wasa) no fat added	2–4 slices ($^3/_4$ oz.)
tortilla chips, no oil added, baked, 0 grams fat	7
pretzels, fat-free, 0 grams fat	12
zweibach	3 ($^3/_4$ oz.)
rice cakes, 4" across	2

---

*3 grams or more of fiber per serving.

Dried Beans, Peas, and Lentils

beans and peas (cooked) such as kidney,
split, white, blackeye, pinto, and garbanzo . . . $^1/_2$ cup
lima beans . . . . $^2/_3$ cup
*lentils (cooked) . . . . $^1/_2$ cup
miso . . . . 3 Tbsp.

Starchy Vegetables

baked beans (no pork, canned). . . . . $^1/_3$ cup
*corn . . . . $^1/_2$ cup
*corn on the cob, large . . . . $^1/_2$ cob (5 oz.)
peas, green. . . . . $^1/_2$ cup
parsnips . . . . $^2/_3$ cup
*peas, green (canned or frozen) . . . . $^1/_2$ cup
potato (white), boiled . . . . $^1/_2$ cup or
$^1/_2$ medium (3 oz.)
potato (mashed) . . . . $^1/_2$ cup
potato, baked with skin. . . . . $^1/_4$ large (3 oz.)
jicama (cooked). . . . . $^3/_4$ cup
*succotash . . . . $^1/_3$ cup
sweet potato, yam, plain . . . . $^1/_2$ cup
squash, winter (acorn, butternut,
pumpkin) . . . . $^1/_2$ cup
*plantain . . . . $^1/_2$ cup

Starch Foods Prepared with Fat—Count the following as 1 starch/bread choice + 1 fat choice

croutons. . . . . 1 cup
biscuit, $2^1/_2$" across 1
popover . . . . 1 average

---

*3 grams or more of fiber per serving

Starch Foods Prepared with Fat (cont.)

refried beans . . . . ½ cup

taco shell, 5" across 2

chow mein noodles . . . . ½ cup

crackers, round butter type 6

french fried potatoes, 2" to 3½" long . . . . . 10 (1½ oz.)

fried rice . . . . ⅓

muffin, plain, small 1

pancake, 4" across 2

stuffing, bread (prepared) . . . . ⅓ cup

waffle 4" square 1

whole wheat crackers, fat added (such
as Triscuits) . . . . 4–6 (1 oz.)

hummus . . . . ⅓ cup

sandwich crackers, cheese or peanut
butter filling 3

snack chips (potato, tortilla) . . . . 9–13 (¾ oz.)

Fruit choices

One fruit choice contains 15 grams of carbohydrate and 60 calories (weights include skin, core, seeds, and rind).

Fruits are valuable sources of vitamins, minerals, and fiber. Fresh, frozen, and dried fruits have about 2 grams of fiber per serving. Fruits that have 3 or more grams of fiber per serving are marked with a * symbol in the list. Fruit juices contain very little fiber.

Vitamin C is abundant in citrus fruits and juices and is found in raspberries, strawberries, mangoes, cantaloupe, honeydews, and papayas. The better sources of vitamin A among these fruits are fresh or dried apricots, mangoes, cantaloupe, nectarines, yellow peaches, and persimmons. Many fruits are valuable sources of potassium—apricots, bananas, several types of berries, grapefruit, grapefruit juice, mangoes, cantaloupe, honeydews, nectarines, oranges, orange juice, and peaches.

Fruits from the list may be fresh, dried, canned, frozen, cooked, or raw, as long as no sugar is added. Whole fruit is more filling than fruit juice and so may be a better choice for those who are trying to lose weight. When drinking juice, it is better to include it with your meals.

One choice is equal to:

$^1/_2$ cup of fresh fruit or fruit juice

$^1/_4$ cup of dried fruit

1 small to medium fresh fruit

Fruit

apple, fresh . . . . 1 small or $^1/_2$ medium
(4 oz.)

apples, dried . . . . 4 rings

apple slices, spiced . . . . $^1/_2$ cup

applesauce. . . . . $^1/_2$ cup

apricots, fresh . . . . 4 whole (5 $^1/_2$ oz.)

apricots, canned . . . . $^1/_2$ cup

*apricots, dried . . . . 8 halves

banana, small . . . . 1 (4 oz.)

Berries:

*blackberries, raw. . . . . $^3/_4$ cup

blackberries, cooked or canned . . . . $^3/_4$ cup

*blueberries. . . . . $^3/_4$ cup

boysenberries . . . . $^3/_4$ cup

loganberries. . . . . $^3/_4$ cup

---

*3 grams or more of fiber per serving

Fruit (*cont.*)

raspberries, cooked, canned, or raw . . . . . 1 cup

*strawberries, raw, whole . . . . $1^{1}/_{4}$ cup

strawberries, cooked or canned . . . . $1^{1}/_{4}$ cup

cantaloupe, small . . . . 1 cup cubes (11 oz.)

casaba melon. . . . . $^{1}/_{10}$

cherries, sweet, fresh. . . . . 12 (3 oz.)

cherries, sweet, canned. . . . . $^{1}/_{2}$ cup

citrus sections . . . . $^{3}/_{4}$ cup

dates 3

*figs, fresh or dried. . . . . $1^{1}/_{2}$ large

fruit cocktail . . . . $^{1}/_{2}$ cup

grapefruit, canned, sections . . . . $^{3}/_{4}$ cup

grapefruit, fresh. . . . . $^{1}/_{2}$ small (11 oz.)

grapes, fresh, small . . . . 17 (3 oz.)

guava . . . . 1 small

honeydew, cubed. . . . . 1 cup

kiwi . . . . 1 ($3^{1}/_{2}$ oz.)

kumquat . . . . 3–4 medium

mandarin orange, canned . . . . $^{3}/_{4}$ cup

mango . . . . $^{1}/_{2}$ small ($5^{1}/_{2}$ oz.)

mixed fresh fruit . . . . $^{1}/_{2}$ cup

*nectarine, small. . . . . 1 (5 oz.)

orange, canned, sections. . . . . $^{1}/_{2}$ cup

orange, fresh . . . . 1 small ($6^{1}/_{2}$ oz.)

papaya, cut up. . . . . 1 cup

peaches, canned . . . . $^{1}/_{2}$ cup

peach, fresh. . . . . 1 medium (4 oz.)

pears, canned . . . . $^{1}/_{2}$ cup

pear, fresh, large . . . . $^{1}/_{2}$ (4 oz.)

---

*3 grams or more of fiber per serving

Fruit (cont.)

persimmons.	2 medium
pineapple, canned	$^1/_2$ cup
pineapple, fresh, cut up	$^3/_4$ cup
pineapple coleslaw	$^1/_2$ cup
plums, fresh, 2" across	2 small
*pomegranate	1 small
*prunes, stewed or dried	3 medium
raisins	2 Tbsp.
tangelos	1 medium
tangerines, small	2 (8 oz.)
tropical fruit salad	$^1/_4$ cup
watermelon	$1^1/_4$ cup, 1 slice ($13^1/_2$ oz.)

Fruit Juice, Unsweetened

apple juice/cider	$^1/_2$ cup
cranberry juice cocktail	$^1/_3$ cup
cranberry juice cocktail, reduced-calorie . . .	1 cup
fruit juice blends, 100% juice	$^1/_3$ cup
grape juice	$^1/_3$ cup
grapefruit juice	$^1/_2$ cup
lemon juice	$^3/_4$ cup
lime juice	$^1/_2$ cup
orange juice	$^1/_2$ cup
pineapple juice	$^1/_2$ cup
prune juice	$^1/_3$ cup
low carb juices	1 cup
(sugar free, light style)	

---

*3 grams or more of fiber per serving

Milk choices

One milk choice contains 12 grams of carbohydrate and 8 grams of protein.

This list contains different types of milk and milk products. Cheeses are on the meat lists, and cream and other dairy fats are on the fat choice list.

The amount of fat in milk is measured in percent (%) of butterfat. The calories in dairy products vary depending on what kind of milk is used in them.

Milk is a rich source of protein, calcium, and riboflavin (a B vitamin). You can use the milk allowed in your meal plan either to drink, on cereal, or in cooking. Look for chocolate milk, rice milk, frozen yogurt, and ice cream on the other carbohydrate choice lists.

One serving of each of the three types of milk (fat-free/low-fat, reduced-fat, and whole) includes the following:

	Carbohydrate (grams)	Protein (grams)	Fat (grams)	Calories
fat-free/low-fat ($^1/_2$% or 1%)	12	8	0–3	90
reduced-fat (2%)	12	8	5	120
whole	12	8	8	150

One milk choice is equal to:

1 cup milk

$^3/_4$ cup yogurt

Fat-Free Milk (0–3 grams fat per serving)

fat-free milk . . . . 1 cup
$1/2$% milk . . . . 1 cup
1% milk. . . . . 1 cup
Buttermilk, low-fat or fat-free. . . . . 1 cup
Evaporated fat-free milk. . . . . $1/2$ cup
Dry fat-free milk. . . . . $1/3$ cup
Lactaid 100, fat-free . . . . 1 cup
Soy milk, low-fat or fat-free . . . . 1 cup
Yogurt, plain fat-free . . . . $3/4$ cup (6 oz.)
Yogurt, fat-free, flavored,
sweetened with nonnutritive
sweetener and fructose. . . . . $3/4$ cup (6 oz.)

Reduced-Fat Milk (5 grams fat per serving)

Reduced-fat milk (2%) . . . . 1 cup
Yogurt, plain low-fat . . . . $3/4$ cup (6 oz.)
Sweet acidophilus milk. . . . . 1 cup
Lactaid 100 reduced-fat milk . . . . 1 cup
Soymilk. . . . . 1 cup

Whole Milk (8 grams fat per serving)

Whole milk. . . . . 1 cup
Evaporated whole milk. . . . . $1/2$ cup
Goat's milk . . . . 1 cup
Kefir . . . . 1 cup
Yogurt, plain (made from whole milk) . . . . . 1 cup (8 oz.)

Other carbohydrate choices

You can use food choices from the list below for a starch, fruit, or milk choice on your meal plan. Some choices will also count as one or more fat choices. Moderate amounts of these foods can be used in your meal plan even if they do contain sugar or fat, as long as you maintain blood sugar control. Check with your dietitian as to how often you can plan them in your diet. Remember to always check the nutrition facts on the food label, which will be your best source of information.

One choice equals 15 grams carbohydrate, or 1 starch, 1 fruit, or 1 milk.

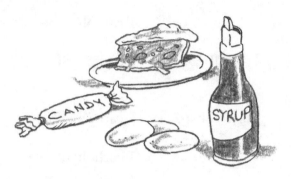

Food	Serving Size	Choices per Serving
angel food cake, unfrosted	1/12th full size cake	2 carbohydrates
brownie, small unfrosted	2" square	1 carbohydrate, 1 fat
cake, unfrosted	2" square	1 carbohydrate, 1 fat
cake, frosted	2" square	2 carbohydrates, 1 fat
cookie, fat-free	2 small	1 carbohydrate
cookie or sandwich cookie with creme filling	2 small	1 carbohydrate, 1 fat
cupcake, frosted	1 small	2 carbohydrates, 1 fat
cranberry sauce, jellied	$1/4$ cup	2 carbohydrates
croissant	1 petite	1 carbohydrate, 2 fats
craisins	$1/2$ ounce	1 carbohydrate
doughnut, plain cake	1 medium ($1\frac{1}{2}$ oz.)	$1\frac{1}{2}$ carbohydrates, 2 fats

Food	Serving Size	Choices per Serving
doughnut, glazed	$3^3/_4$" across (2 oz.)	2 carbohydrates, 2 fats
energy, sport, or breakfast bar	1 bar ($1^1/_2$ oz.)	$1^1/_2$ carbohydrates, 0–1 fat
fruit juice bars, frozen, 100% juice	1 bar (3 oz.)	1 carbohydrate
fruit snacks, chewy (pureed fruit concentrate)	1 roll ($^3/_4$ oz.)	1 carbohydrate
fruit spreads, 100% fruit	$1^1/_2$ Tbsp.	1 carbohydrate
gelatin, regular	$^1/_2$ cup	1 carbohydrate
gingersnaps	3	1 carbohydrate
ice cream	$^1/_2$ cup	1 carbohydrate, 2 fats
ice cream, light	$^1/_2$ cup	1 carbohydrate, 1 fat
ice cream, low-fat	$^1/_2$ cup	$1^1/_2$ carbohydrates
ice cream, fat-free, no sugar added	$^1/_2$ cup	1 carbohydrate
jam or jelly, regular	1 Tbsp.	1 carbohydrate
milk, chocolate, whole	1 cup	2 carbohydrates, 1 fat
pie, fruit, 2 crusts	$^1/_6$ pie	3 carbohydrates, 2 fats
pie, pumpkin or custard (commercially prepared)	$^1/_8$ pie	2 carbohydrates, 2 fats
potato chips	12–18 (1 oz.)	1 carbohydrate, 2 fats
pudding, regular (made with low-fat milk)	$^1/_2$ cup	2 carbohydrates
pudding, sugar-free (made with fat-free milk)	$^1/_2$ cup	1 carbohydrate

Food	Serving Size	Choices per Serving
reduced calorie meal replacement (shake)	1 can (10–11 oz.)	$1^1/_2$ carbohydrates, 0–1 fat
rice milk, low-fat or fat-free, plain	1 cup	1 carbohydrate
rice milk, low-fat, flavored	1 cup	$1^1/_2$ carbohydrates
salad dressing, fat-free	$^1/_4$ cup	1 carbohydrate
sherbet, sorbet	$^1/_2$ cup	2 carbohydrates
spaghetti or pasta sauce, canned	$^1/_2$ cup	1 carbohydrate, 1 fat
sports drinks	8 oz. (1 cup)	1 carbohydrate
sweet roll or Danish	1 ($2^1/_2$ oz.)	$2^1/_2$ carbohydrates, 2 fats
syrup, light	2 Tbsp.	1 carbohydrate
syrup, regular	1 Tbsp.	1 carbohydrate
syrup, regular	$^1/_4$ cup	4 carbohydrates
tortilla chips	6–12 (1 oz.)	1 carbohydrate, 2 fats
vanilla wafers	5	1 carbohydrate, 1 fat
yogurt, frozen, fat-free	$^1/_3$ cup	1 carbohydrate
yogurt, frozen	$^1/_2$ cup	1 carbohydrate, 0–1 fat
yogurt, low-fat, with fruit	1 cup	3 carbohydrates, 0–1 fat

Always check label. Products may vary.

Vegetable choices

One vegetable choice contains 5 grams of carbohydrate, 2 grams of protein, 0 grams of fat, 2–3 grams of fiber, and 25 calories.

Vegetables that contain small amounts of carbohydrates and calories are on this list. Vegetables have a lot of very important nutrients. Include two to three choices in your meal plan each day. Starchy vegetables such as corn, peas, potatoes, and winter squash that contain large amounts of carbohydrates and calories are on the starch choice list.

Dark-green and deep-yellow vegetables are among the leading sources of vitamin A. Many of the vegetables in the starch group are good sources of vitamin C—asparagus; broccoli; brussels sprouts; cabbage; cauliflower; collards; dandelion, mustard, and turnip greens; kale; rutabagas; spinach; tomatoes; and turnips.

Moderate amounts of vitamin B6 are supplied by broccoli, Brussels sprouts, cauliflower, collard greens, sauerkraut, spinach, tomatoes, and tomato juice.

Good sources of potassium include broccoli, Brussels sprouts, beet and chard greens, tomatoes, tomato juice, and vegetable juice cocktails.

If fat is added in cooking these vegetables, it must be counted from your allowed fat choices.

When using cooked vegetables, figure that one pound of most raw vegetables yields about $4^1/_2$ cups. One pound of cooked spinach or kale yields 8 to $12^1/_2$ portions.

One vegetable choice is equal to:

$^1/_2$ cup of cooked vegetables or vegetable juice

1 cup of raw vegetables

If you eat only one or two vegetable choices at a meal or snack, you do not have to count them, because they contain only small amounts of calories and carbohydrates.

artichoke globe	beets
artichoke hearts	bok choy
asparagus	broccoli
bamboo shoots	Brussels sprouts
beans (green, wax, Italian)	cabbage (red/green)
bean sprouts	carrots

cauliflower

celery

chayote

cucumber

eggplant

green onions or scallions

greens (all—beet, chard, collard, dandelion, kale, mustard, spinach, turnip)

jicama

kohlrabi

leeks

mixed vegetables (without corn, peas, or pasta)

mushrooms

okra

onions

pea pods (including Chinese)

peppers (all varieties)

pimiento

radishes

rhubarb

rutabaga

salad greens (endive, escarole, lettuce, romaine, spinach)

sauerkraut

summer squash

tomatoes (fresh whole)

tomato/vegetable juice

tomato paste

tomato puree

tomato sauce

tomatoes, canned

turnips

water chestnuts

watercress

zucchini

Meat or Meat Substitute Choices

One average meat choice contains 7 grams of protein.

All of the foods in the meat list are good sources of protein, and many are also good sources of iron, zinc, vitamin B12 (present only in foods of animal origin), and other B vitamins.

Meats take a major part of the food budget, but more importantly they are high in calories, saturated fat, and cholesterol. Using more lean and very lean meat, poultry, and fish in your meals will help reduce your risk of heart disease. Meats in the high-fat group should be limited to 3 servings a week.

Buy only what you plan to eat. As a guide, allow about one-quarter weight loss in cooking—for 1 pound of raw meat allow for a loss of 4 ounces, leaving 12 ounces of cooked meat (see page 90).

Be sure to trim off all visible fat from meats. Use a non-stick pan spray or a nonstick pan to sauté or brown foods. If you flour or bread your meat, count it as a starch serving in your meal plan. Meat juices with the fat removed may be used with your meat or vegetables for added flavor without counting them as an added serving.

The following lists are divided into four sections: very lean, lean, medium-fat, and high-fat. They are based on the amount of fat and calories in one serving, or one ounce, of meat.

	Carbohydrate	*Protein*	*Fat*	*Calories*
very lean	0 grams	7 grams	0–1 gram	35
lean	0 grams	7 grams	3 grams	55
medium-fat	0 grams	7 grams	5 grams	75
high-fat	0 grams	7 grams	8 grams	100

One meat choice is equal to:

1 oz. meat, fish, poultry, or cheese

$^{1}/_{2}$ cup dried beans

Very lean meat and substitutes
One choice equals 0 grams carbohydrate, 7 grams protein, 0–1 gram fat and 35 calories. One very lean meat choice is equal to any one of the following:

Poultry

chicken or turkey (white meat, no skin), ... 1 oz.
Cornish hen (no skin)

Fish

fresh or frozen cod, flounder, haddock, halibut, ... 1 oz.
trout, lox (smoked salmon); tuna, fresh or canned in water

Shellfish

clams, crab, lobster, scallops, shrimp, ... 1 oz.
imitation shellfish

Game

duck or pheasant (no skin), venison, buffalo, ostrich . . . 1 oz.

Cheese with 1 Gram or Less Fat per Ounce

low-fat cottage cheese . . . . $^1/_4$ cup
fat-free cheese . . . . 1 oz.

Other

processed sandwich meats with 1 gram or less fat . . . . . . 1 oz.
per ounce, such as deli thin, shaved meats,
chipped beef, turkey ham
egg whites 2
egg substitutes, plain . . . . $^1/_4$ cup
hot dogs with 1 gram or less fat per ounce . . . . 1 oz.
kidney (high in cholesterol) . . . . 1 oz.
sausage with 1 gram or less fat per ounce . . . . 1 oz.

Count as one very lean meat and one starch choice:

dried beans, peas, lentils (cooked) . . . . $^1/_2$ cup

Lean meat and substitutes

One choice equals 0 grams carbohydrate, 7 grams protein, 3 grams fat, and 55 calories. One lean meat choice is equal to any one of the following:

Beef

USDA select or choice grades of lean beef trimmed . . . . . 1 oz.
of fat, such as round, sirloin, and flank steak;
tenderloin; roast (rib, chuck, rump); steak
(T-bone, porterhouse, cubed), ground round

Pork

lean pork, such as fresh ham; canned, cured, or . . . . 1 oz.
boiled ham; Canadian bacon; tenderloin, center
loin chop

Lamb

roast, chop, leg . . . . 1 oz.

Veal

lean chop, roast . . . . 1 oz.

Poultry

chicken, turkey (dark meat, no skin), chicken . . . . 1 oz.
(white meat, with skin), domestic duck or goose
(well drained of fat, no skin)

Fish

herring (smoked, not creamed) . . . . 1 oz.
oysters . . . . 6 medium
salmon (fresh or canned), catfish . . . . 1 oz.
sardines (canned) . . . . 2 medium
tuna (canned in oil, drained) . . . . 1 oz.

Game

goose (no skin), rabbit . . . . 1 oz.

Cheese

4.5%-fat cottage cheese . . . . $^1/_4$ cup
grated Parmesan . . . . 2 Tbsp.
cheeses with 3 grams or less fat per ounce . . . .•. . . . . 1 oz.

Other

hot dogs with 3 grams or less fat per ounce . . . . $1^1/_2$ oz.
processed sandwich meat with 3 grams or less fat
per ounce, such as turkey pastrami or kielbasa . . .
liver, heart (high in cholesterol) . . . . 1 oz.

Medium-fat meat and substitutes
One choice equals 0 grams carbohydrate, 7 grams protein, 5 grams fat, and 75 calories. One medium-fat choice is equal to any one of the following:

Beef

most beef products (ground beef, meatloaf,
corned beef, short ribs, prime grades of
meat trimmed of fat, such as prime rib). . . . . .1 oz.

Pork

top loin, chop, Boston butt, cutlet . . . . 1 oz.

Lamb

rib roast, ground . . . . 1 oz.

Veal

cutlet (ground or cubed, unbreaded) . . . . 1 oz.

Poultry

chicken dark meat (with skin), ground
turkey or chicken, fried chicken (with skin) . . . . .1 oz.
turkey bacon. . . . . 2 slices

Fish

Any fried fish product . . . . 1 oz.

Cheese with 5 Grams or Less Fat per Ounce

feta . . . . 1 oz.

mozzarella . . . . 1 oz.

ricotta . . . . $^{1}/_{4}$ cup (2 oz.)

Other

egg (high in cholesterol, limit to 3 per week) 1

sausage with 5 grams or less fat per ounce . . . . 1 oz.

tempeh . . . . $^{1}/_{4}$ cup

tofu . . . . 4 oz. or $^{1}/_{2}$ cup

edamame . . . . $^{1}/_{2}$ cup

High-Fat Meat and Substitutes

One choice equals 0 grams carbohydrate, 7 grams protein, 8 grams fat, and 100 calories.

Remember that these items are high in saturated fat, cholesterol, and calories and may raise blood cholesterol levels if eaten on a regular basis. One high-fat meat choice is equal to any one of the following:

Pork

spareribs, ground pork, pork sausage . . . . 1 oz.

Cheese

all regular cheeses, such as American,
cheddar, Monterey Jack, Swiss. . . . . 1 oz.

Other

processed sandwich meats with 8
grams or less fat per ounce, such as
bologna, pimento loaf, salami. . . . . 1 oz.

sausage, such as bratwurst, Italian,
knockwurst, Polish, smoked. . . . . 1 oz.

hot dog (turkey or chicken) 1 (10/lb.)

bacon . . . . 3 slices (20 slices/lb.)

peanut butter (contains unsaturated fat) . . . . 1Tbsp.

Count as one high-fat meat plus one fat exchange:

hot dog (beef, pork, or combination) 1 (10/lb.)

Fat Choices

One fat choice contains 5 grams of fat and 45 calories.

Fats come from both animal and vegetable sources and range from liquid oils to hard fats. Oils are fats that remain liquid at room temperature and are usually from a vegetable source. Common vegetable oils are olive, peanut, corn, soybean, canola, and sunflower oils. Common animal fats are butter, cream, and bacon fat. All fats are high in calories, so foods on this list should be measured carefully to control your weight. Try to include more monounsaturated and polyunsaturated fats in your diet—they are good for your health. Saturated fats and Trans fats in your diet can raise your blood level of cholesterol (see the section "Saturated Fat and Cholesterol," pages 99–101).

One fat choice is equal to:

1 teaspoon of regular margarine or vegetable oil

1 tablespoon of regular salad dressing

The following is a list of foods to use for one fat choice.

Monounsaturated Fats (use these)

avocado, medium . . . . 2 Tbsp. (1 oz.)

oil (canola, olive, peanut) . . . . 1 tsp.

olives:

   ripe black . . . . 8 large

   green stuffed . . . . 10 large

nuts:

   almonds, cashews . . . . 6 nuts

   mixed (50% peanuts) . . . . 6 nuts

   peanuts . . . . 10 nuts

   pecans . . . . 4 halves

peanut butter, smooth or crunchy . . . . $^1/_2$ Tbsp.

sesame seeds . . . . 1 Tbsp.

tahini or sesame paste . . . . 2 tsp.

Polyunsaturated Fats (use these)

margarine:

   stick, tub, or squeeze . . . . 1 tsp.

   lower-fat (30% to 50% vegetable oil) . . . 1 Tbsp.

mayonnaise:

   regular . . . . 1 tsp.

   reduced-fat . . . . 1 Tbsp.

oil (corn, safflower, soybean) . . . . 1 tsp.

nuts: English walnuts . . . . 4 halves

salad dressing:

   regular . . . . 1 Tbsp.

   reduced-fat . . . . 2 Tbsp.

Miracle Whip salad dressing:

   regular . . . . 2 tsp.

   reduced-fat . . . . 1 Tbsp.

seeds: pumpkin, sunflower, pine nuts . . . . 1 Tbsp.

Saturated Fats (avoid)

bacon	1 slice (20 slices/lb.)
bacon grease	1 tsp.
butter:	
stick.	1 tsp.
whipped	2 tsp.
reduced-fat	1 Tbsp.
chitterlings, boiled	2 Tbsp.
chocolate, unsweetened	2 tsp.
coconut, sweetened, shredded	2 Tbsp.
coconut milk.	1 Tbsp.
cream, half and half	2 Tbsp.
cream cheese:	
regular.	1 Tbsp. ($^{1}/_{2}$ oz.)
reduced-fat	$1^{1}/_{2}$ Tbsp. ($^{3}/_{4}$ oz.)
cream: heavy, whipping	1 Tbsp.
sour cream:	
regular.	2 Tbsp.
reduced-fat	3 Tbsp.
salt pork	1 oz.
shortening or lard.	1 tsp.

Note: Nondairy creamers, powdered or liquid, are not included on these food lists (see the free food list on page 68). These products differ in food value, but usually 1 tablespoon provides about 20 calories (mainly in the form of carbohydrate). In powdered form, 2 teaspoons have 20–25 calories, including 2 grams of carbohydrate and less than 1 gram of fat. Try using 1 teaspoon of nonfat dry milk in your coffee. It costs less and only has 10 calories per teaspoon.

Combination Foods

Most of the meals we eat contain different kinds of foods mixed together. It is hard to fit these in any one list, so we grouped them together. It is often hard to tell what is in a casserole or prepared food item. With carbohydrate counting it is easier to fit these combination foods such as soups and frozen dinners into your meal plan. Remember to look at the grams of starch or carbohydrate, protein, and fat listed on the package Nutrition Facts label. Ask your dietitian about favorite foods you would like to include in your meal plan.

Food Items	Measure	Food Choices
Entrees		
casseroles, homemade	1 cup (8 oz.)	2 carbohydrates 2 med.-fat meats
cheese pizza, thin crust	$^1/_4$ of 15-oz. or $^1/_4$ of 10"	2 carbohydrates 2 med.-fat meats 1 fat
chili with beans	1 cup (8 oz.)	2 carbohydrates 2 med.-fat meats
lasagna	3" × 4"	2 carbohydrates 2 med.-fat meats
chow mein without rice or noodles	2 cups (16 oz.)	1 carbohydrate 2 lean meats
Soups		
instant with beans/lentils	1 cup (8 oz.)	$2^1/_2$ carbohydrate 1 very lean meat
cream (made with water)	1 cup (8 oz.)	1 carbohydrate 1 fat
split pea (made with water)	$^1/_2$ cup (4 oz.)	1 carbohydrate
tomato (made with water)	1 cup (8 oz.)	1 carbohydrate
vegetable beef, chicken noodle, or other broth type	1 cup (8 oz.)	1 carbohydrate

Food Items	Measure	Food Choices
Frozen Entrees (items are light or low-calorie)		
creamy garlic shrimp	1 package 11.5 ounces 270 calories	2 starch 2 very-lean meats 1 vegetable
chicken Teriyaki	1 package 11 ounces 260 calories	2 starch 2 very-lean meats 1 vegetable
country glazed chicken	1 package 8.5 ounces 230 calories	2 starch 2 very-lean meats
cheesy glazed chicken	1 package 9.5 ounces 260 calories	2 starch 2 lean meats
turkey breast and mashed potatoes	1 package 8.5 ounces 210 calories	1½ starch 2 lean meats
manicotti	1 package 11 ounces 290 calories	2½ starch 1 lean meat 1 vegetable
three cheese ziti marinara	1 package 9 ounces 290 calories	3 starch 2 med.-fat meats 1 fat

Free Foods List

Some food items are called *free foods*. This is a food or drink that contains less than 20 calories a serving and has 5 grams or less of carbohydrate per serving. Limit "free foods" to 3 servings per day divided between meals and snacks. When a food or drink contains more than 5 grams of carbohydrate, always count it in your meal plan.

When using the following free foods, use only the amount shown.

A-1 Sauce . . . . 1 Tbsp.
catsup . . . . 1 Tbsp.
chili sauce . . . . 1 Tbsp.
cocoa (dry, unsweetened powder) . . 1 Tbsp.
cranberries. $^1/_3$ cup cooked without
sugar
cream cheese, fat-free . . . . 1 Tbsp.
creamer, light nondairy, liquid . . . . . 2 Tbsp.
creamer, nondairy, liquid . . . . 1 Tbsp.
creamer, nondairy, powdered . . . . . . 2 tsp.
hard candy, sugar-free . . . . 1 candy
jam or jelly, low-sugar or light . . . . . 2 tsp.
margarine, fat-free. . . . . 4 Tbsp.
margarine, reduced-fat . . . . 1 tsp.
mayonnaise, fat-free . . . . 1 Tbsp.
mayonnaise, reduced-fat . . . . 1 tsp.
Miracle Whip, nonfat . . . . 1 Tbsp.
Miracle Whip, reduced-fat . . . . 1 tsp.
Nestlé Quik, sugar-free . . . . 1 heaping Tbsp.
pickles, dill . . . . $1^1/_2$ large
pickle relish. . . . . 1 Tbsp.
pickles, sweet (bread and butter) . . . 2 slices
pickles, sweet (gherkin) . . . . $^3/_4$ oz.
salad dressing, fat-free. . . . . 1 Tbsp.
salad dressing, fat-free Italian . . . . . . 2 Tbsp.
salad spritzers . . . . 10 sprays
salsa. . . . . $^1/_4$ cup
sauerkraut juice . . . . 1 cup
sour cream, fat-free, reduced-fat. . . . 1 Tbsp.
soy sauce. . . . . 1 Tbsp.
syrup, sugar-free . . . . 2 Tbsp.
taco hot sauce . . . . 1 Tbsp.
whipped topping, regular or light . . 2 Tbsp.
Worcestershire sauce. . . . . 1 Tbsp.
yeast (brewer's) . . . . 2 tsp.
yogurt (plain) . . . . 2 Tbsp.

What is the Healthy Diabetes Plate

The healthy Diabetes Plate takes the five food groups and helps you see what *healthy meals* looks like. All you need is a 9-inch plate for your vegetable choices, starch choices, meat and meat substitute choices, plus a small bowl and a glass for your fruit choice and milk choice.

You don't need any special tools or have to do any counting. It's easy to draw an imaginary line down the middle of your plate. Then on one side, divide it again so have three sections on your plate.

- The plate method will help you:
- Eat a variety of foods from all food groups.
- Control how much you eat (your portion sizes).
- Control your blood sugar.

Here is how to make a meal using the Plate Method.

1. Fill 1/2 of your plate with vegetable choices such as broccoli, cauliflower, green beans, and salad.

2. Fill 1/4 of your plate with a meat or meat substitute choice such as chicken or fish; about 3 ounces.

3. Fill 1/4 of your plate with a starchy choice such as 1/3 cup of rice or pasta.

4. A one fruit choice 1 small apple or 1 cup of cubed honeydew.

5. Choose one milk choice such as 1 cup of nonfat or lowfat milk, or 3/4 cup yogurt.

6. Add margarine or oil for preparation or add at the table.

7. Add 1 free food if desired.

8. For breakfast, use only half the plate. 1/4 of your plate is from the meat or meat substitute choices list. The other 1/4 is from the starch choice list. You can also have 1 fruit choice and 1milk choice depending on your meal plan.

Lunch and Dinner

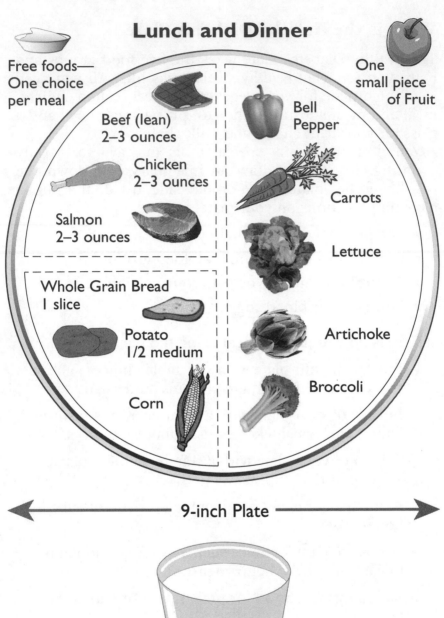

Free foods—
One choice
per meal

Beef (lean)
2–3 ounces

Chicken
2–3 ounces

Salmon
2–3 ounces

Whole Grain Bread
1 slice

Potato
1/2 medium

Corn

Bell
Pepper

Carrots

Lettuce

Artichoke

Broccoli

One
small piece
of Fruit

← 9-inch Plate →

One cup (8 ounces)
of lowfat or nonfat
Milk

	Morning Meal	**Noon Meal**	**Evening Meal**
Carbohydrate choices			
Starch			
Fruit			
Milk/Yogurt			
Vegetable			
Meat/Protein			
Fat			
Generally For women: 2–3 servings (30–45 grams)			
Carbohydrate choices (PER MEAL)			
For men: 3–4 servings (45–60 grams)			
Carbohydrate choices (PER MEAL)			

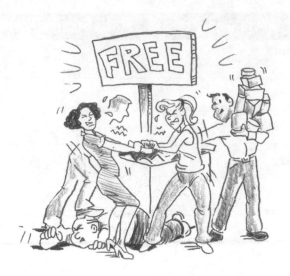

When using spreadable 100% fruit products that look and spread like jam, limit your serving to 1 teaspoon.

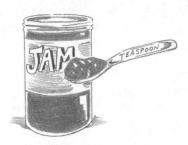

The following list includes items that are sugar-free and low-calorie that can be used in your meal plan as much as you want:

Drinks

bouillon, broth, consommé

club soda

drink mixes, sugar-free

soft drinks, sugar-free

tonic water, sugar-free

tea or coffee

Condiments
lime juice
mustard
Pam vegetable spray
vinegar

Sugar-free items
alternative sweeteners
gelatin (unflavored)
gelatin dessert
gum
soft drinks

Seasonings are also free foods. You may use any amount of the following in your meal plan:

allspice	cumin
angostura bitters	curry
anise	dill
basil	extracts (vanilla, etc.)
bay leaf	garlic
caraway	ginger root
cardamom	mace
celery salt or seed	marjoram
chervil	mint
chili powder	monosodium glutamate
chives	mustard, dry
cinnamon	nutmeg
cloves	oregano

Seasonings (*continued*)

paprika	saffron
parsley	sage
pepper	sesame seed
poppy seed	tenderizers
poultry seasoning	thyme
rosemary	

Snacks

Do you need snacks? This will depend on several things such as:

1. Are you a "grazer" and like to eat several times throughout the day?
2. Your type of diabetes medicine/s
3. How many hours are there between your meals
4. Exercise/activity—amount and timing

Here are some examples of snacks divided into three groups. Discuss your need for snacks and what foods the snacks should contain with your diabetes educator (dietitian or nurse).

1. **Snacks where there are more than 4–5 hours between meals or BEDTIME.** This snack should contain 1 serving of carbohydrate + 1 serving of protein.

   Examples: 1/2 sandwich
   1 serving of crackers + peanut butter
   1 corn tortilla + low-fat cheese
   sugar-free yogurt + nuts
   1 serving crackers + string cheese
   1/2 English muffin + peanut butter
   1 serving crackers + cottage cheese
   1 fruit serving + nuts
   1 fruit serving + string cheese

2. **Snacks when there are LESS than 4–5 hours between meals, but do have calories so be careful of the amounts.**

   Examples: 1 serving of a sugar-free item such as 1/2 cup
   pudding or ice cream
   1 serving sugar-free cookies
   1 sugar-free fudge bar
   1 serving sugar-free candies
   nuts or seeds
   1 serving of a protein food such as 1 oz. meat,
   1 string cheese, 1/2 cup cottage cheese
   vegetables

3. Free foods. These foods contain less than 5 grams or less of carbohydrate.

   Examples: sugar-free jello or popsicles, diet drinks, coffee, tea, water, sugar-free flavored waters.

Dietetic Foods

Be cautious about any type of dietetic food. Although they are lower in sugar, dietetic foods often contain other foods that break down into sugar. Be extra careful of dietetic ice cream, cookies, candy bars, cakes, and so on, because many of these products contain more calories than the foods they are replacing.

Learn to read Nutrition Facts labels (see pages 84–87) and know the nature of the product you are buying. An item labeled "dietetic" may not be right for someone with diabetes. It could contain less sugar, less salt, less fat, or less cholesterol than the regular product.

You need to read the label to find out why it claims to be dietetic, and you need to decide whether you really need it. For example, dietetic cookies may be sugar-free but still contain flour, fat, and calories from alternative sweeteners that must be counted in your daily meal plan.

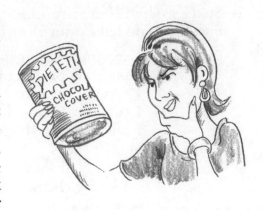

Alternative Meals and Snacks

There are supplements available that can be used by anyone with diabetes. They are available in liquid shakes and bars. They can be used as a meal replacement, a snack, or during an illness as long as they are part of your meal plan. There are several products available. Always check labels.

Example:

Glucerna drink	Glucerna bar
Vanilla 8 ounces	Lemon crunch
220 calories	1 bar 140 calories
1 starch	$1\frac{1}{2}$ starch
1 low-fat milk	$\frac{1}{2}$ fat
1 fat	
Choice drinks	Choice bar
Vanilla 8 ounces	Fudge Brownie
220 calories	1 bar 140 calories
1 starch	1 starch
1 low-fat milk	1 fat
2 fats	

SAMPLE MEAL PLANS

The following are sample meal plans for calorie levels 1,500 and 2,000. Use them only as a temporary guide, and check with your doctor or dietitian for more complete meal plans suited to your personal needs (timing, snacks, and medication) and tastes.

The meal plan on page 78 is blank. (Extra forms are included at the back of the book.) It will be used by your dietitian when planning your personal meal plan. She or he will determine the total carbohydrate, meat, and fat choices for one day based on your calorie needs.

Using the same form, plan several of your own menus. Examples have been provided to use as guides. First, though, go back to the choice lists on pages 43–68 and mark all the foods you like to eat for breakfast, lunch, dinner, and snacks. Take notice of the amount of those foods that equal one choice. Then plan your meals to fit your meal plan.

Example: If you are on a 1,500-calorie meal plan and at breakfast you are allowed 3 carbohydrate choices, one day you may choose:

$1/2$ cup cereal

$1/2$ banana

1 cup fat-free milk

or

1 small bagel

$1/2$ grapefruit

When choosing other foods, you can choose within the same food group, but do not switch a starch food for a meat food. You can also add free foods, as long as you stay within the guidelines for your meal plan.

Personalized Meal Plan

Number of Calories _____
Carbohydrate: _____ grams   Protein: _____ grams
Fat: _____ grams

Breakfast Time: _____

_____ Carbohydrate Choices
  _____ starch
  _____ fruit
  _____ milk
_____ Meat Choices
_____ Fat Choices

Morning Snack Time: _____
_____

Lunch Time: _____

_____ Carbohydrate Choices
  _____ starch
  _____ fruit
  _____ milk
_____ Vegetables
_____ Meat Choices
_____ Fat Choices

Afternoon Snack Time: _____
_____

*Dinner Time:*_____

_____ Carbohydrate Choices
  _____ starch
  _____ fruit
  _____ milk
_____ Vegetables
_____ Meat Choices
_____ Fat Choices

Evening Snack Time: _____
_____

Sample Meal Plan
1,500 Calories

Sample Menu

Breakfast

3 carbohydrate choices:
  1 starch $^1/_2$ cup bran cereal
  1 fruit $^1/_2$ banana
  1 fat-free milk   1 cup fat-free milk
1 very lean meat $^1/_4$ cup reduced-fat cottage cheese

Lunch

4 carbohydrate choices:
  2 starches   2 slices wheat bread
  1 fruit   1 small apple
  1 fat-free milk   1 cup fat-free milk
vegetable   carrot sticks, lettuce, and tomato
2 very lean meat choices   2 oz. sliced turkey (white meat)
1 fat choice   1 Tbsp. reduced-fat mayonnaise

Dinner

4 carbohydrate choices:
  3 starches   1 cup wild rice
  1 fruit $^1/_2$ cup fresh fruit
vegetable $^1/_2$ cup green beans
                   lettuce salad with tomato
2 lean meat choices   2 oz. baked chicken (no skin)
2 fat choices   1 tsp. margarine
                   2 Tbsp. reduced-fat
                   dressing
                   iced tea (no sugar)

Bedtime Snack

1 starch   1 slice wheat toast
1 lean meat choice   1 oz. low-fat cheese

Sample Menu

Breakfast

4 carbohydrate choices:

2 starches	1 English muffin
1 fruit	$^1/_2$ grapefruit
1 fat-free milk	1 cup fat-free milk
1 fat choice	1 tsp. margarine
1 med.-fat meat choice	1 poached egg

Morning Snack

1 carbohydrate choice	$^3/_4$ cup plain fat-free yogurt

Lunch

4 carbohydrate choices:

3 starches	1 cup vegetable beef soup
	2 slices wheat bread
1 fruit	17 small fresh grapes
vegetable	lettuce and tomato
2 lean meat choices	2 oz. sliced turkey (white meat)
1 fat choice	1 Tbsp. reduced-fat mayonnaise
	sugar-free soft drink

Afternoon Snack

1 starch choice	6 saltine crackers
1 lean meat choice	1 oz. string cheese

Dinner

5 carbohydrate choices:

3 starches	1 cup mashed potatoes
	1 small wheat roll
1 fruit	$1^1/_4$ cups whole strawberries
1 starchy vegetable	$^1/_2$ cup green peas
vegetable	lettuce salad
3 lean meat choices	3-oz. grilled salmon

2 fat choices	2 Tbsp. reduced-fat dressing
	1 tsp margarine
free drink	iced tea (no sugar)

Bedtime Snack

| 1 starch | $^1/_2$ bagel, small |
| 1 protein | 1 Tbsp. peanut butter |

ALTERNATIVE SWEETENERS

There are three types of sweeteners: caloric, noncaloric, and those that are half and half. Caloric sweeteners such as sucrose (table sugar) contain about 16 calories per teaspoon. Sweeteners labeled low calorie, or lite, are $^1/_2$ sugar and $^1/_2$ noncaloric sweetener, and contain 8 calories per teaspoon. There are five noncaloric sweeteners on the market. They contain a very small amount of carbohydrate, sugar, or calories and will give you the sweet taste of sugar but will not raise blood glucose levels. You will find these sweeteners in diet soda, diet gelatin, chewing gum, fruit drinks, and powdered drink mixes. As long as the serving has less than 20 calories and less than 5 grams of carbohydrate per serving you can use it as a free food. When using noncaloric sweeteners in beverages and other food items, 1 packet is usually equal to 2 tsp. sugar.

In the following chart, noncalorie sweeteners are compared.

Aspartame–(NutraSweet, Equal) is used to sweeten many foods and beverages. Not recommended for baking because prolonged exposure to heat will cause loss of sweetness.

Sucralose–(Splenda) is the sweetest noncaloric sweetener available. It can be used in cooking and baking and is also used as the sweetening in many foods and beverages.

Saccharin–(Sweet'n Low, Sugar Twin) has been used for many years. It can be used in cooking, baking, canning, or sprinkled on cereals or fruit. Saccharin may have a bitter aftertaste to some people.

Acesulfame-K–(Sweet One, Sunett) may also have a bitter aftertaste to some people. It can be used in coffee and tea and on cereal and fruits. It is used in combination with other noncaloric sweeteners in many low-calorie, sugar-free and no-added-sugar foods.

Stevia–(Truvia) comes from a plant leaf and is used in other food and beverages.

Sugar Alcohols

Some low calorie or no-added-sugar foods replace sucrose with sugar alcohols. These are carbohydrates that have a lower calorie level than other carbohydrates. They provide 2 calories per gram per serving compared to 4 calories per gram. They are absorbed more slowly than sucrose and cause a smaller rise in blood glucose.

Sugar alcohols will be listed on the Nutrition Facts label and added in as part of the total carbohydrate. If the total carbohydrate in the food comes from sugar alcohols and there is less than 5 grams per serving, it can be counted as a free food. If a food contains more than 5 grams of sugar alcohol, subtract half the grams of sugar alcohol from the grams of carbohydrate to get the available carbohydrate grams. The remaining carbohydrate needs to be figured into your meal plan. Products that may use sugar alcohols are low calorie candies, cookies, chewing gum, drinks, pudding, and sugar-free cough drops.

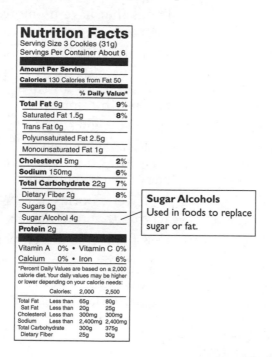

Nutrition Facts

Serving Size 3 Cookies (31g)
Servings Per Container About 6

Amount Per Serving

Calories 130 Calories from Fat 50

	% Daily Value*
Total Fat 6g	9%
Saturated Fat 1.5g	8%
Trans Fat 0g	
Polyunsaturated Fat 2.5g	
Monounsaturated Fat 1g	
Cholesterol 5mg	2%
Sodium 150mg	6%
Total Carbohydrate 22g	7%
Dietary Fiber 2g	8%
Sugars 0g	
Sugar Alcohol 4g	
Protein 2g	

Vitamin A   0% • Vitamin C 0%
Calcium   0% • Iron   6%

*Percent Daily Values are based on a 2,000 calorie diet. Your daily values may be higher or lower depending on your calorie needs:

		Calories: 2,000	2,500
Total Fat	Less than	65g	80g
Sat Fat	Less than	20g	25g
Cholesterol	Less than	300mg	300mg
Sodium	Less than	2,400mg	2,400mg
Total Carbohydrate		300g	375g
Dietary Fiber		25g	30g

Sugar Alcohols
Used in foods to replace sugar or fat.

UNDERSTANDING FOOD LABELS

In 1993 the United States Food and Drug Administration (FDA) created Nutrition Facts labels. This label can be useful to you in making HEALTHIER FOOD CHOICES. To help you understand the food labels, the FDA has explained the terms used on them, for example, *light, calorie-free, low-fat, high-fiber,* and *low-cholesterol.*

The following information will help you to understand these terms and serve as a guide you can use when you are choosing foods.

Term	Meaning
Calorie free	Less than 5 calories per serving.
Reduced calorie	Has at least 25% fewer calories than the regular food but is equal in food value.
Low calorie	Foods that have no more than 40 calories per serving.
Diet, dietetic	Term used for both low-calorie and reduced-calorie foods. May also be used on foods low in sodium but not low in calories.
Artificially sweetened	Same as reduced-calorie or low-calorie, except that sucrose (table sugar) has been removed and alternative sweetener added.
Light, lite	$1/3$ fewer calories or 50% less fat per serving than the regular food.
Fat-free	Less than $1/2$ gram fat per serving.
Low-fat	3 grams or less fat per serving.
Reduced-fat	At least 25% fewer calories than the regular food.

Term	Meaning
High fiber	5 grams per serving.
More or added fiber	2.5 grams or more per serving than the regular food.
Low in saturated fat	1 gram or less saturated fat per serving. No more than 15% of the calories are from saturated fat.
Cholesterol-free	Less than 2 milligrams cholesterol per serving.
Low cholesterol	Less than 20 milligrams cholesterol and less than 2 grams saturated fat per serving.
Sodium-free, salt-free	Less than 5 milligrams sodium per serving.
Low sodium	Less than 140 milligrams sodium per serving.
Enriched, fortified	Foods must contain 10% more of Daily Value for protein, vitamins, minerals, dietary fiber, or potassium per serving.
No added sugar, Without added sugar No sugar added	Permitted if no sugars or ingredient that substitutes for sugars is used, contains no fruit juice concentrate or jelly.

How to Read a Food Label

Nutrition Facts on a food label can help you with food choices.

Serving sizes are based on what people usually eat. Check your meal plan to see if the amount equals your food choices.

Calories per serving and *calories* per serving *from fat* are listed.

% daily value can be used to compare foods and see how the amount of a nutrient in a serving of food fits into a 2,000-calorie-per-day diet.

The nutrient list covers the information important in helping you make HEALTHY FOOD CHOICES.

- *Total fat* shows the amount in one serving. One fat choice has 5 grams of fat. If the label reads 10 grams of fat, a serving will count as 2 fats in your meal plan. The amount of saturated fat and Trans fat is shown

- *Cholesterol* shows how a serving of this compares with the recommended 300 milligrams of cholesterol each day.

- *Sodium* shows how a serving of this food compares with the recommendation of 2,400 milligrams of sodium each day.

- *Total carbohydrate* is more important to look at than just sugar content. One starch, fruit, milk, or other carbohydrate has about 15 grams of carbohydrate. If the label reads 30 grams, a serving will count as 2 starch choices. Dietary fiber is found under total carbohydrate.

- *Protein* tells you the number of meat choices in a serving. One meat choice has 7 grams of protein. If the label reads 14 grams of protein, a serving will count as 2 meat choices.

Vitamins and minerals: Manufacturers only have to list vitamins A and C and minerals, calcium, and iron. The amounts are a percentage of the USRDA (recommended daily allowances).

Fiber shows how this food compares with the recommendation of 25 grams of fiber per day.

% daily value gives a general idea of how much fat, sodium, carbohydrate, or dietary fiber a serving provides to your daily diet. Use it to find foods low in fat and high in fiber.

Calories per gram gives you the number of calories in a gram each of fat, carbohydrate, and protein.

Nutrition Facts

Serving Size ½ cup (11—g)
Servings Per Container 1

Amount Per Serving

Calories 90	Calories from Fat 30
	% Daily Value*
Total Fat 3g	5%
Saturated Fat 0g	0%
Trans Fat 0g	
Cholesterol 0mg	0%
Sodium 300mg	13%
Total Carbohydrate 13g	4%
Dietary Fiber 3g	12%
Sugars 3g	
Protein 3g	

Vitamin A	80%	• Vitamin C	60%
Calcium	4%	• Iron	4%

* Percent Daily Values are based on a 2,000 calorie diet. Your daily values may be higher or lower depending on your calorie needs:

		2,000	2,500
Total Fat	Less than	65g	80g
Sat Fat	Less than	20g	25g
Cholesterol	Less than	300mg	300mg
Sodium	Less than	2,400mg	2,400mg
Total Carbohydrate		300g	375g
Fiber		25g	30g

Calories per gram:
Fat 9   •   Carbohydrate 4   •   Protein 4

Serving sizes are stated in both household and metric measures and reflect the amounts people actually eat.

Calories from fat are now shown on the label to help consumers meet dietary guidelines that recommend people get no more than 30 percent of their calories from fat.

The list of nutrients covers those most important to the health of today's consumers, most of whom need to worry about getting *too much* of certain items (fat, for example) rather than too few vitamins or minerals, as in the past.

Remember: It is more important to look at the *total carbohydrate* content on a food label than the amount of sugar.

ALCOHOL

Many times the question is asked, "What about alcohol—can I have a drink once in a while?" There is no set answer to this question. Much depends on your blood sugar control, weight, and blood fat levels. Therefore, **discuss the use of alcohol with your doctor.** If you do decide to use alcohol, you must fully understand how to do so properly in your meal plan. To assist you, here are some facts you need to know.

- Alcohol is absorbed quickly and has 7 calories per gram.
- Alcohol has no food value.
- Alcohol is burned differently than food by your body and does NOT require insulin to be used.
- Alcohol may cause hypoglycemia (low blood sugar), especially if you take diabetes pills or insulin and meals are missed or delayed (it prevents the body from putting new glucose or sugar into the blood from storage sites in the liver).
- If taken by someone on Diabinese (see pages 120–121), alcohol may cause a reaction such as flushing, sweating, headache, nausea, or a choking sensation.
- Avoid alcohol if your triglycerides are high or you are taking Glucophage-Metformin.
- Avoid alcohol if you must lose weight—alcohol provides calories and can stimulate the appetite.

Suggestions for the Use of Alcohol

- If individuals choose to drink alcohol, daily intake should be limited to one drink for adult women and two drinks for adult men. One drink is defined as 12 oz. beer, 5 oz. wine, or 1.5 oz. of hard liquor (a shot).

■ Alcohol can lower your blood sugar, so use it only with meals and snacks. Taking alcohol with meals slows down its absorption into the bloodstream and "smooths out" its effect on the body.

■ Avoid sweet wines, liqueurs, and sweetened mixed drinks because of their high sugar content. Mixers such as orange juice must be counted in your total calorie count.

How to Plan for Alcohol in Your Diet

Alcohol runs through the body like fat and must be counted as a fat choice. One fat choice should be removed for every 45 calories in the alcoholic drink. Refer to the chart below for calorie content:

liquor	gin, vodka, rum, whiskey 1 oz. = 70 calories
dry wine	chablis, chianti, champagne 3 oz. = 60 calories
beer (low-calorie)	12 oz. = approximately 70 to 100 calories
beer (regular)	12 oz. = 171 calories

COOKING with alcohol: Alcohol evaporates at about 172°F, which is below the simmering stage. The flavor of the beverage is left, but the calories and the alcohol are lost.

REMEMBER: Discuss the use of alcohol with your doctor.

SHOPPING TIPS

Plan your menus for a week at a time, taking advantage of grocery store specials. Make a shopping list of the items you need according to their location in the store. Pick up dairy, cold, and frozen items last. Also, to avoid overeating, estimate the quantity of foods you need to buy.

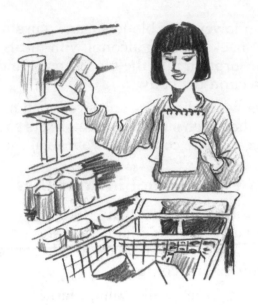

Example: For a family of two adults and two children less than 12 years old (if 12 years or older, treat as an adult):

For each child: 3 oz. (before cooking) meat × 2 = 6 oz.

For each adult: 4 oz. (before cooking) meat × 2 = 8 oz.

Amount meat needed for a meal = 14 oz.

If, in the above example, you cooked 2 pounds of chicken, you should have about 1 pound of meat left over to be used in another meal (sandwiches, tacos, stews, etc.).

DINING OUT IN RESTAURANTS

To make it easier to stick to your meal plan, use the following suggestions on foods you should or should not order in a restaurant.

Do Order

Appetizers	Vegetable juices and soups; unsweetened and fresh fruit juices; fresh fruit cocktails; clear broth, bouillon, or consommé; fresh vegetables, salads, celery, radishes, dill pickles, lettuce, or tomato (all without dressing added). Ask for vinegar and oil, French, or Italian dressing on the side.
Meat, fish, poultry	Roasted, baked, broiled, boiled, or grilled. Trim off extra fat. Order fish, chicken, or turkey rather than beef or pork.
Potatoes	Mashed, baked, boiled, or steamed potatoes, plain tortillas, steamed rice, or plain noodles. When served with butter, count as a fat choice.
Vegetables	Stewed, steamed, or boiled. When served with butter, count as a fat choice.
Breads	Any kind of bread of average thickness. Order hard or soft rolls. A small plain muffin, biscuit, or cornbread may be used but must be counted as 1 starch and 1 fat choice.
Fats	Margarine, mayonnaise, salad dressing, or avocado. Use only amounts allowed in your meal plan.
Desserts	Fresh fruits; sponge, angel food, or pound cake; plain vanilla ice cream. Remember to count all items in your meal plan.
Beverages	Coffee, tea, fat-free or reduced-fat milk, vegetable juices, or sugar-free drinks.

Do Not Order

Appetizers	Creamed soups, sweetened juices, canned fruit cocktail, salads with dressing already added (except coleslaw or potato or pasta salad).
Meat, fish, poultry	Fried, sautéed, stewed, braised, breaded, or in a casserole. Foods served with gravy or in a sauce.
Potatoes	Home-fried, French-fried, browned, creamed, scalloped.
Vegetables	Creamed, scalloped, au gratin, fried, or sautéed.
Breads	Sweet rolls, coffee cake, frosted or sweetened breads. Fried tortillas.
Fats	Gravy, fried foods, foods with cream sauces such as creamed chicken.
Desserts	Rich desserts, pies, or pastries.
Beverages	Regular soft drinks, chocolate milk, cocoa, milk drinks such as milk shakes.

Suggestions to Help Make Restaurant Meals Easier for You

- Memorize your meal plan so you can substitute foods at a glance from the menu.
- Measure foods at home so that you can judge portion sizes in restaurants.
- When you see foods with special names on the menu (for example, Chicken Supreme), ask the waiter what is in the dish or how it is made.
- Restrict the number of restaurants you go to as much as possible—you will become familiar with their menus,

and the waiters may remember how you want your food prepared.

■ Don't make a habit of eating everything on your plate. If portion sizes are too large, take home what is left in a take-out bag.

■ Be on the lookout for fats. By planning ahead you can save fat choices from earlier in the day for the meal you will be eating out.

■ Ask for sauces, gravy, and dressing on the side so that you can use less than is normally served with a dish.

■ Think about the timing of your meals. If you take a medication for your diabetes, having meals on time is critical for preventing hypoglycemia. When your meal is delayed more than one hour, have 1 carbohydrate choice (starch, fruit, milk) while you wait. If you need to take insulin before the meal, take it with you.

What about Fast Foods?

Contrary to popular belief, fast foods can be nutritious. If wise choices are made, fast food can fit into your meal plan once in a while.

Avoid large orders of high-fat foods such as double cheeseburgers with French fries. Be aware of the high-fat sauces added to sandwiches and of the hidden fats in fried foods (onion rings, deep-fried zucchini, etc.). When ordering a baked potato, avoid a lot of fat and calories by topping your potato with vegetables, chives, or spices rather than cheese sauce, bacon, and sour cream.

Most fast-food chains now offer a variety of salads. Use low-calorie, light, or reduced-calorie salad dressing. Avoid prepared salads such as potato or pasta salad. Never order foods high in sugar, such as fruit pies, cookies, ice cream, sundaes, and milk shakes. Order diet soft drinks rather than regular ones. Be aware that such foods as fish sandwiches, fried chicken pieces, and fried and barbecued chicken sandwiches may appear healthy but can be high in calories, fat, and sodium.

Here are some tips to help you choose well when ordering food choices to fit into your meal plan:

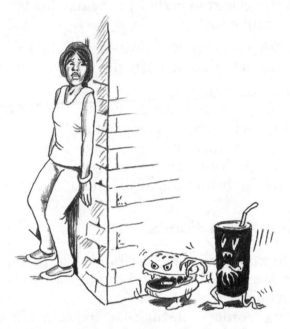

- Know that the average fast-food meal contains about 685 calories. It is not too high for a meal, but it is too high in calories for a snack.

- If you are having fast food for one meal, have your other meals that day contain healthier foods, such as fruits and vegetables.

- Choose grilled or broiled sandwiches with meats such as lean roast beef, turkey or chicken breast, or lean ham. Order items plain or with mustard and lettuce.

- Avoid croissants. Eat your sandwich on a bun or wheat bread to save calories and fat.

- Order tacos, tostados, bean burritos, soft tacos, and other nonfried items when eating Mexican fast food. Choose chicken over beef. Avoid beans refried in lard. Use extra lettuce, tomatoes, and salsa instead of cheese, sour cream, or guacamole.

- Pizza is a good fast-food choice. Order thin-crust pizza with vegetable toppings.

- When ordering sandwiches your best choice is a regular or junior size instead of the deluxe size.

- Use mustard instead of mayonnaise or mayonnaise-based dressing. This will save you about 100 calories per tablespoon.

- If breakfast is your fast-food meal, choose a plain small bagel, toast, a fat-free muffin, or an English muffin. Order plain scrambled eggs or pancakes without butter.

Fast-Food Choices for Your Meal Plan

Food	Serving Size	Calories	Choices
Burger King			
Hamburger	1	330	2 starch 2 med.-fat meats
Chicken Tenders	5 pieces	220	1 starch 1 med.-fat meat 1 fat
Broiled Chicken Salad Red. Cal. Lt. Italian	1	200	2 vegetables 3 very lean meats 1 fat

Fast-Food Choices for Your Meal Plan (*cont.*)

Food	Serving Size	Calories	Choices
McDonald's			
Hamburger	1	260	2 starch 2 med.-fat meats
Bacon Ranch Salad with Grilled Chicken	1	260	4 lean meats 1 starch
Grilled Chicken Classic Sandwich	1	420	2 starch 4 lean meats
In-n-Out Burger			
Hamburger *with mustard and catsup instead of spread	1	390	$2^1/_2$ starch 2 med.-fat meats 2 fats
Wendy's			
Junior Hamburger	1	280	2 starch 1 high-fat meat
Grilled Chicken Sandwich	1	370	3 starch 3 lean meats
Broccoli and Cheese baked potato	1	340	4 starch 1 vegetable
Jack in the Box			
Chicken Fajita Pita	1	290	2 starch 3 med.-fat meats
Asian Chicken Salad	1	140	1 starch 2 med.-fat meats
Hamburger	1	310	2 starch 2 med.-fat meats 3 fats

Fast-Food Choices for Your Meal Plan (*cont.*)

Food	Serving Size	Calories	Choices
Taco Bell			
Taco	1	170	$1^1/_2$ starch 1 med.-fat meat
Tostado	1	250	2 starch 1 med.-fat meat
Soft Chicken	1	190	1 starch 1 med.-fat meat
Baja Fresh			
Baja-style Taco with Chicken	1	190	$1^1/_2$ starch 1 lean meat
Shrimp Ensalada	1	180	$^1/_2$ starch 2 vegetables 2 lean meats 1 fat
Baja style Taco with Steak	1	220	$1^1/_2$ starch 1 lean meat 1 fat
Rubio's			
Health Mex Chicken Taco	1	170	$1^1/_2$ starch 2 lean meats
Health Mex Chicken Salad	1	260	2 starch 3 lean meats
Subway			
Veggie Delight Sandwich	1 small	230	$2^1/_2$ starch 1 lean meat 1 vegetable
Turkey Breast Sandwich	1 small	280	$2^1/_2$ starch 2 lean meats 1 vegetable

Fast-Food Choices for Your Meal Plan (*cont.*)			
Food	Serving Size	Calories	Choices
Subway			
Turkey Sandwich	6", small	280	3 starch 2 lean meats 1 vegetable
Pizza Hut			
Thin Crust Cheese	2 slices	400	3 starch 2 med.-fat meats 2 fats
Starbucks			
Caffe Latte (nonfat)	12oz.	120	1 fat-free milk
Cappuccino (nonfat)	12oz.	80	1 fat-free milk
Coffee Frappuccino	12 oz.	200	$2^1/_2$ starch $^1/_2$ fat

REMEMBER: When you decide to eat fast food, be sure you balance your meal plan by eating vegetables, fruits, fat-free milk, and whole-grain foods at your other meals.

For more information on fast foods, you can write or check the Web sites of the following restaurants:

Burger King Corporation
   Consumer Information M/S 1441
   P.O. Box 520783
   General Mail Facility
   Miami, FL 33152
   www.burgerking.com

McDonald's Corporation
   Consumer Affairs
   2111 McDonald's Drive
   Oak Brook, IL 60523
   www.mcdonalds.com

Carl's Jr.
  Carl Karcher Enterprises
  1200 N. Harbor Blvd.
  Anaheim, CA 92803
  www.carlsjr.com

El Pollo Loco (Denny's)
  3333 Michelson
  Irvine, CA 92612
  www.elpolloloco.com

In-n-Out Burger
  4199 Campus
  Irvine, CA 92612
  www.in-n-out.com

Jack In The Box
  9330 Balboa Ave.
  San Diego, CA 92123
  www.jackinthebox.com

KFC
  Consumer Affairs Dept.
  P.O. Box 32070
  Louisville, KY 40232
  www.kfc.com

Pizza Hut, Inc.
  Consumer Affairs Dept.
  P.O. Box 428
  Witchita, KS 67201
  www.pizzahut.com

Rubios
  Corporate Office
  1902 Wright Place
  Carlsbad, CA 92008
  www.rubios.com

Subway
  325 Bic Drive
  Medford, CT 06460
  www.subway.com

Taco Bell
  17901 Von Karman
  Irvine, CA 92714
  (800)TACO BELL
  www.tacobell.com

Wendy's International, Inc.
  Consumer Affairs Dept.
  P.O. Box 256
  Dublin, OH 43017
  www.wendys.com

SATURATED FAT AND CHOLESTEROL

It is recommended that people with diabetes lower saturated fat intake to less than 10% of calories and eliminate Trans fats in their diet. Dietary cholesterol should be limited to 300 milligrams cholesterol per day. If your LDL cholesterol is too high, individuals may be told to lower their saturated fat intake to 7% of calories and limit their cholesterol intake to 200 milligrams per day.

Diabetes and Blood Fat Goals

HDL ("good") cholesterol	Greater than 40 mg/dl for men, Greater than 50 mg/dl for women
LDL ("bad") cholesterol	Less than 100 mg/dl
Total Cholesterol	Less than 200 mg/dl
Triglycerides	Less than 150 mg/dl

Fats You Eat

Diets that are high in saturated fat have been shown to raise blood cholesterol levels. This in turn can increase your risk of heart and blood vessel disease.

The majority of fat in your diet should be in the form of monounsaturated and polyunsaturated fat. These fats raise the HDL cholesterol and lower LDL cholesterol. They come from plants and include oils that are liquid at room temperature, for example, nuts, seeds, and canola, cottonseed, sunflower, soybean, olive, peanut oils and margarine. Choose margarine that has a liquid oil, such as olive oil or soybean oil, as its first ingredient rather than a partially hydrogenated oil or Trans fat.

Saturated fat raises blood cholesterol (total cholesterol and LDL), plus your own body makes a large part of the cholesterol found in your blood. Saturated fats are found in animal fats, meats, solid shortenings, some vegetable oils (palm, coconut oils, and cocoa butter), whole milk dairy products (cheese and butter). If your blood fats are high, your doctor may prescribe medicine that will help lower them, but you will still want to follow your specific meal plan.

Trans fats are produced when liquid oil is made into a solid fat through a process called hydrogenation. Trans fats act like saturated fats and can raise your cholesterol levels. In 2006 Trans fats are to be listed on nutrition labels and ingredient lists. Many snack foods like crackers, chips and processed baked goods have Trans fats as well as fast-food items like French fries.

Guidelines to Help Reduce the Amount of Fat and Cholesterol in Your Meal Plan

- Use fish, chicken, turkey, and veal in most of your meat-containing meals for the week. Look for names like loin, round, lean, choice and select.
- Trim all visible fat from meats and skin from poultry before cooking.
- Avoid deep-fat frying. Cook with methods that remove fat (baking, broiling, barbecuing, etc.).
- Select fat-free or reduced-fat products when buying luncheon meats, baked goods, salad dressings, dairy products and baked goods.
- Avoid gravies, sauces, and creamy casserole dishes.
- Limit egg yolks to four per week, including those used in cooking.
- Use a nonstick cooking spray on pans and utensils.

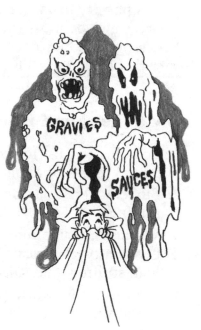

- Check labels on "sugar free" cookies and desserts. They may be sugar free, but more than 60 percent of their calories can come from fat.
- Check the meat or meat substitute choices (very lean & lean meat) list on pages 57–61 for meat choices that are lower in fat.

FIBER IN YOUR DIET

What is fiber? It is not a vitamin or a mineral, it does not contain calories, and it is an important part of your diet.

There are different types of fiber that do different things for your body. Some hold water; others affect the absorption of nutrients. When fiber holds water it is acting like a sponge in your body, absorbing water and making the gut contents bulkier. When you eat fiber, it softens your stools, and they can be passed with less effort.

Fiber is good for treating or preventing stomach and intestinal problems, including colon cancer. A large amount of fiber helps to keep blood fats (cholesterol and triglycerides) lower.

The intake of fiber for people with diabetes should be the same as for those without diabetes.

> Your daily amount of fiber intake should be 20 to 35 grams per day from a large selection of foods. Good sources include most fruits, vegetables, whole grains, seeds, nuts, and legumes (beans). We suggest that you include high-fiber foods in your meal plan every day.

How to Eat More Fiber

1. Look for cereals that contain "whole grain" and have at least 3 grams of dietary fiber per serving.
2. Buy crackers that contain 2 grams of dietary fiber per serving.
3. Work some high fiber foods like nuts, bulgur or wheat germ into your meals. Mix them with casseroles, meat loaf, stuffing, and salads.
4. Choose whole-wheat pasta, brown rice, and any whole-wheat version for other foods you eat.
5. Add any type of beans, corn, or peas to your meal plan for your starch choices.

Counting the Fiber

When there is enough fiber, it will change how you count the total carbohydrate in the food. When a starch food has more than 5 grams of fiber, you subtract $1/2$ the fiber from the total amount of carbohydrate.

EXAMPLE

40 grams Total Carbohydrate
− 5 grams Fiber
35 grams Total Carbohydrate

25 grams Total Carbohydrate
−$3^1/2$ grams Fiber
$21^1/2$ grams Total Carbohydrate

Nutrition Facts

Serving Size: 1 cup (55 g)
Servings per container: about 7

Amount Per Serving

	Cereal	Cereal + 125 ml of skim milk
Calories	190	230
Calories from fat	20	25
	% Daily Value*	
Total Fat 2.5g	4%	4%
Saturated Fat 0g	0%	0%
Trans Fat 0g		
Cholesterol 0 mg	0%	0%
Sodium 200 mg	8%	11%
Total Carbohydrate 40g	13%	15%
Dietary Fiber 10g	40%	40%
Sugars 16g		
Protein 8g		2%
Vitamin A	0%	4%
Vitamin C	2%	2%
Calcium	25%	40%
Iron	15%	15%
Folic Acid	100%	100%
Vitamin b-12	110%	110%

Total Fat	Calories:	2,500	2,500
Total Fat	Less Than	65g	80g
Sat Fat	Less Than	20g	25g
Cholesterol	Less Than	300mg	300mg
Sodium	Less Than	2,400mg	2,400mg
Total Carbohydrate		300g	375g
Dietary Fiber		25g	30g

Calories per gram:
Fat 9 • Carbohydrate 4 • Protein 4

Nutrilion Facts

Serving Size: 1 Bagel 2 oz. (57g)
Servings Per Container: 5

Amount Per Serving

Calories 110	Calories from fat 0
	% Daily Value*
Total Fat 0g	0%
Saturated Fat 0 g	0%
Trans Fat 0 g	
Cholesterol 0 mg	0%
Sodium 210 mg	9%
Total Carbohydrate 25 g	8%
Dietary Fiber 7g	
Sugars 0g	
Protein 6g	

Vitamin A	0%	•	Vitamin C	0%
Calcium	15%	•	Iron	8%

*Percent Daily Values are based on a 2,000 calorie diet. Your daily values may be higher or lower depending on your calore needs:

		Calories	2,000	2,500
Total Fat	Less Than		65g	80g
Sat Fat	Less Than		20g	25g
Cholesterol	Less Than		300mg	300mg
Sodium	Less Than		2,400mg	2,400mg
Total Carbohydrate			300g	375g
Dietary Fiber			25g	30g

Calories per gram:
Fat 9 • Carbohydrate 4 • Protein 4

The following lists will give you some ideas on how to add high-fiber foods to your meal plan.

Fruits		
Good Sources		*Poor Sources*
apricots (dried)	applesauce	apple juice
apples (with skin)	apricots	grape juice
blackberries	(fresh/canned)	orange juice
blueberries	bananas	pineapple juice
cranberries	cherries	
figs (dried)	grapefruit	
papayas	mango	
passion fruit	plum, small	
pears	nectarines	
pomegranates	oranges	
prunes	peaches	
raspberries	kiwi	
strawberries		
tangerine, small		

Vegetables		
Good Sources		*Poor Sources*
artichoke	asparagus	tomato juice
beets	cabbage	
broccoli	carrots	
brussels sprouts	cauliflower	
sauerkraut	celery	
	cucumbers	
	eggplant	
	lettuce	

Vegetables (cont.)

Good Sources		Poor Sources
parsnips	tomatoes	
turnip greens	spinach	
soybeans	squash (zucchini)	
string beans		

Starches, Grains, and Legumes

Good Sources		Poor Sources
rye wafer crackers	bulgur	bread, white
cooked beans	shredded wheat	noodles
(kidney, pinto,	wild rice	saltines
black, white)	corn, cooked	Rice Krispies
green peas, frozen,	popcorn	puffed rice
boiled	tortillas	animal crackers
lima beans	(corn, wheat)	pretzels
dried beans, peas,	potatoes	rice, white
lentils	(white with skin)	
squash (winter, acorn,	sweet potatoes	
and butternut)	Triscuits	
bran cereal (All Bran	reduced fat	
Bran Buds,	wheat germ,	
Fiber One)	toasted	
cereals with	multigrain pasta	
greater than	chickpeas	
5 grams of	corn	
fiber	cowpeas	

Nuts, Seeds, and others

Good Sources		Poor Sources
sunflower seeds	coconut	
pumpkin seeds	nuts (cashews, almonds,	
sesame seeds	pecans, hazelnuts,	
	peanuts)	

Sample Meal Plan for a High-Fiber Diet

Breakfast	Lunch	Dinner
blueberries	tuna sandwich on	roast beef
bran flakes	whole-wheat bread	brown rice
poached egg	vegetable soup	dinner salad
whole-wheat bread	celery sticks	broccoli
margarine	strawberries	fresh apple with skin
fat-free milk		whole-wheat bread
		margarine

Evening Snack
rye wafer crackers
peanut butter

MEAL-PLANNING RESOURCES

When you have diabetes, your diet cannot be short-term just to lose weight or control blood sugar. You must learn an entire new style of eating that you can follow for the rest of your life. Don't be disappointed about giving up favorite foods. Learn how to develop a sense of balance with food. Think of it as changing your old eating habits to new ones. This is not an easy thing to do. It takes time to form new habits.

A good resource if you need help is a registered dietitian (R.D.), an expert in diet and nutrition. To locate a registered dietitian in your area, search "registered dietitian" or visit www.eatright.org. You can also check the Academy of Nutrition and Dietetics. This is a national referral service that allows you to find an R.D. to help you.

References

All references or cookbooks from the American Diabetes Association. Call 1-800-342-2383, or look up www.shopdiabetes.org.

Complete Guide to Carb Counting, 3rd edition, by Hope Warshaw BC-ADM, RD CDE, and Karmeen Kulkami, MS, RD, CDE. American Diabetes Association, 2011.

- Includes basic and advanced carb counting in meals and using food levels. It includes an appendix of everyday foods, 2011.

Eat What You Love, Love What You Eat with Diabetes, by Michelle May, MD, with Megrette Fletcher, MED, RD, CDE. New Harbinger Publications, 2012.

Diabetes Meal Planning Made Easy, 4th edition, by Hope Warshaw, BC-ADM, RD, CDE. American Diabetes Association, 2010.

The Mayo Clinic Diabetes Diet, by the Mayo Clinic Good Books, 2011.

- Helps you stay on track by teaching you helpful tips and tools to improve your diabetes.

Choose Your Foods: Food Lists of Diabetes. American Diabetes Association and Academy of Nutrition and Dietetics, 2014.

The Official Pocket Guide to Diabetic Exchanges, 3rd edition. American Diabetes Association, 2011.

What Can I Eat? The Diabetes Guide to Healthy Food Choices.
American Diabetes Association, 2014.

Journal of the American Dietetic Association Carbohydrate Issues: Type and Amount, by Madelyn L. Wheeler and F. Xavier Pi-Sunyer, April 2008: pages 534–539.

Eat Out, Eat Well, by Hope Warshaw, RD,CDE, MMSc, published by the American Diabetes Association, 2015.

- Includes facts on how to eat out and choose your meals wisely.

What to Eat When You Get Diabetes, by Carolyn Leontos, RD, CDE, Published by John Wiley and Sons, 2000.

- Easy and appetizing ways to make healthy changes in your meals.

The Calorie King, Fat and Carbohydrate Counter, by Allan Borushek, Family Health Publications, Costa Mesa, Calif., new edition annually. www.CalorieKing.com

- Easy to carry pocket-size book. Includes 200 fast-food restaurants.
- Calorie King App.

Complete Meal Ideas—10 Perfect Plates. American Diabetes Association.

Eating Healthy with Diabetes. American Diabetes Association and Academy of Nutrition and Dietetics, 2014.

The Stress Free Diabetes Kitchen by Barbara Seelig-Brown, American Diabetes Association, 2012.

Cookbooks

More Diabetic Meals in 30 Minutes or Less by Robin Webb, MS, 2nd edition. American Diabetes Association, 1999.

- Contains over 200 recipes.
- All recipes are quick and easy.

Mr. Food's Diabetic Dinners in a Dash. American Diabetes Association, 2006.

- Contains over 150 recipes.
- Fast and easy cooking.

Gluten Free Recipes for People with Diabetes by Nancy S. Hughes and Lara Ronddini-Hamilton, RDLDN, CDE. American Diabetes Association, 2013.

Diabetes Carb Control Cookbook by Nancy S. Hughes. American Diabetes Association, 2014.

Betty Crocker's Diabetes Cookbook: Everyday Meals, Easy as 1-2-3. Betty Crocker Editors. John Wiley and Sons, 2003.

- 140 recipes.
- Uses up-to-the-minute food and nutrition information.

Diabetes Cookbook for Dummies, 2nd edition. Alan Rubin, M.D., Chef Denise Sharf, Alison Acerra, R.D., John Wiley and Sons, 2010.

- Tips on how to do well with restaurant or fast food.
- Nutrition information and diabetic exchanges for each recipe.
- A "visual" guide to portion size.
- A restaurant travel guide.

Diabetes and Heart Healthy Cookbook. American Diabetes Association and American Heart Association, 2014.

- Includes low fat, lower carbohydrate dishes.

The Diabetes Holiday Cookbook: Year Round Cooking for People with Diabetes by Carolyn Leontos, Debra Mitchell, and Kenneth Weicker. John Wiley and Sons, 2002.

- More than 100 recipes for the holidays.
- Alternative ingredient choices for low-sodium and alcohol-free diets.
- Menus for 21 holiday celebrations.

The Diabetes Menu Cookbook: Delicious Special Occasion Recipes for Family and Friends, by Kalia Doner and Barbara Scott-Goodman. John Wiley and Sons, 2006.

- 130 recipes for entertaining and special occasions.
- Includes appetizers and drinks, soups and salads, sandwiches, burgers, wraps, main dishes, and desserts.

Month of Meals: Diabetic Meal Planner, 3rd edition. American Diabetes Association, 2010.

- Over 4,500,000 menu combinations.
- Over 600 recipes and snacks
- Calories, carb counts, fat grams, and exchanges/choices

Month of Meals: Meals in Minutes, 3rd Edition, published by the American Diabetes Association, 2002.

Home Blood-Sugar Testing

Home blood-sugar testing has become one of the most helpful tools in diabetes care. Unlike urine sugar testing, blood sugars are a *direct* measurement of your blood sugar level—they provide "right now" information. You know immediately whether your blood sugar is too high, too low, or in your acceptable range (a range agreed on by you and your doctor).

Being able to test your blood sugars at home, work, or school, during exercise, play, travel, or illness, gives a more realistic look at the pattern your blood sugars form over 24 hours, as well as over several days. By studying this pattern, you and your doctor are able to make better decisions about your blood sugar control and make the necessary adjustments in your medication, exercise, or meal plan. Through such adjustments you can maintain very good, or "tight," blood sugar control, which may help to prevent or slow down some of the complications of diabetes (see pages

187–193). ("Tight" control means most of your blood sugars are in or near your normal range most of the time.)

> What is your acceptable blood sugar range?
> If you do not know, see page 28, or discuss it with your doctor or a diabetes educator.

Home blood-sugar testing can be done by anyone with diabetes. It makes no difference whether you take insulin, oral medications, or are controlling your diabetes by diet alone.

Glucose meters are small battery-operated machines that vary in size from as small as a pen to as large as a small calculator and weigh a few ounces. When a special strip is prepared with one drop of blood, a number appears on the meter giving the blood sugar. Most meters read blood sugars from 0–10 mg/dl up to 600 mg/dl. If the blood sugar is under 10 mg/dl, the meter tells you it's low; if it is over 600 mg/dl, the meter tells you it's high. Glucose meters also tell you the condition of the batteries that operate them and turn themselves off after a certain period of time.

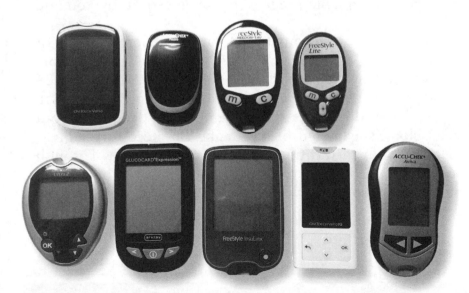

Any glucose meter will provide you with an accurate blood sugar reading if you follow the instructions PRE-CISELY AND CAREFULLY.

In order to test your blood sugar you need one drop of blood, which you obtain by sticking your finger with a small lancet.

Under the round cover is a small, sharp needle.

There are several types of lancet devices that make it easier for you to stick your finger. A lancet is inserted into the lancet device, and a quick spring action provides the finger stick. It also controls how deeply the needle sticks into your finger.

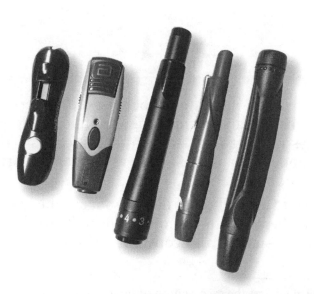

Used lancets are "sharps" and need to be thrown away safely. As the result of a new law in 2008, you can no longer throw them away in the regular garbage. Please turn to page 145 (in the chapter on insulin and syringes) and follow the same steps for throwing away your used lancets.

Helpful hints to remember when testing your blood sugar:

1. Wash your hands carefully and thoroughly with soap and warm water. If you use alcohol,[1] be sure it has dried completely before you stick your finger.

2. Your hand should be warm to increase the blood flow to your fingers. If your hand is cold, warm it by washing it in warm water, rubbing your hands together, or wrapping your hand in a warm wet towel for a few minutes.

3. Stick the side of your finger or thumbtip between the first joint and the very tip.

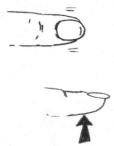

Do not stick your finger behind the fingernail—it is too sensitive and painful there. Some people prefer to always use one area and build up a callus. The callus will not cause any problems, as long as you are able to get a drop of blood.

4. To get a proper drop of blood, squeeze the entire finger from where you finger joins your hand to the fingertip applying smooth and constant pressure.

---

[1] If using alcohol, test the second drop of blood, not the first.

5. Be sure your meter is coded correctly to the code number on the bottle of strips you are using.

6. Check the expiration date on the strips. NEVER use out of date strips. When opening new strips, write the date on the bottle. Once opened, you should finish the bottle within 90 days.

7. Store your glucose meters and strips in cool, dry places. Do not keep them in bathrooms or kitchens or hot cars. They need to be kept under 90 degrees F.

8. Call the 800 phone number on the back of your meter if you have any questions or problems with the meter. There is someone to help you 24 hours every day.

9. WRITE DOWN ALL YOUR BLOOD SUGARS! Record keeping allows you to see PATTERNS in your blood sugars. The numbers will teach you how your blood sugar responds to foods, illnesses, medicines, stress, etc. They will help you make better decisions in food choices and your doctor in diabetes medicine. Take your blood sugar record to your doctor every visit.

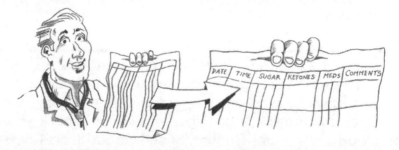

10. Discuss the times you should test your blood sugar with your doctor or diabetes educator. The most helpful testing you can do is a few minutes before AND 2 hours after the start of your different meals.

If all your blood sugar results fall into your acceptable range, then you know your medication, activity, and food are balanced. If results are out of your acceptable range, then you can determine whether there is a pattern to the times when they are high or low. There may be a pattern in the changes in your blood sugar according to the days of the week or the time of day. For example, you may have different blood sugar during the week than on weekends, or your blood sugar may always be high in the afternoon. By seeing these patterns, you and your doctor or diabetes educator can make the necessary changes in food, medication, and/or activity to get your blood sugar into your acceptable range as often as possible.

There are many ways to record your blood sugars. Use the log book that comes with your meter, call the 800 phone number on the back of your meter, or make your own. Use the chart on page 118 as an example. The Comments column is for recording low blood sugar, illness, delayed meals, exercise, emotional stress, or anything else that is affecting your blood sugar (see pages 26–28).

11. When your blood sugars are consistently falling within your acceptable range, you will not need to test as often as when they are out of it. During illnesses or periods of stress you should check your blood sugar more frequently, and, about 3 or 4 days before a visit to the doctor, begin testing more frequently so you have several tests to report.

The more you test, the better control you will have over your blood sugar.

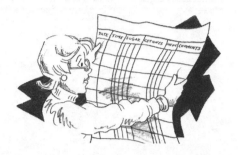

| I WILL TEST MY BLOOD SUGAR: _____ |
| I SHOULD CALL MY DOCTOR WHEN |
| MY SUGAR IS: _____ |

People with diabetes today have a tremendous advantage over those of just a few years ago. Testing blood sugars at home (self-monitoring) has greatly improved one's control over his blood sugar. Now it is possible for you to make medication adjustments depending on the results of your blood sugar tests. Your doctor will give you advice on how and when to make these adjustments.

Remember, good, or "tight," control may prevent, slow down, or lessen some of the long-term complications of diabetes, as well as help you feel your very best. Good control can be achieved by testing your blood sugar and acting on the information—

SO
MAKE
USE
OF IT!

Date	Pre Post Breakfast		Med	Pre Post Lunch		Med	Pre Post Dinner		Med	Bed	Comments

CHAPTER 7

Ketones and Keto-Acidosis

If you have Type 1 diabetes, you will need to test your urine for acetone, or ketones. When there is not enough glucose in the blood (during an insulin reaction) or when there is not enough insulin to allow glucose into the cells, the body looks for a source of energy other than glucose— the other source is fats. As fats are broken down, energy is produced, but you have a waste product called acetone, or ketones.

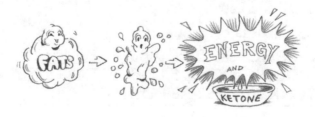

The ketones travel through the blood and are taken out of the body in the urine. Ketones in the urine are a warning that your body is not working properly. Your blood sugar will be high and your urine sugar will be 1 to 2% when your ketones are positive. If this is not quickly corrected it can lead to DIABETIC KETO-ACIDOSIS, which is very serious.

During an insulin reaction, there is not enough sugar to burn for energy, so your body will again break down fat. During this time, your blood sugar will be low and your urine sugar will be negative, but ketones may be positive.

TEST FOR KETONES WHEN[1]

■ your blood sugar is over 250 mg/dl

■ your blood sugar has increased over the past 12 to 24 hours

■ you are ill

■ you think you may have had an insulin reaction but your blood sugar is not low (a positive test for ketones would mean a reaction)

■ urine sugar is 2% or greater

CALL YOUR DOCTOR WHEN

■ your blood sugar is higher than 250 mg/dl and the ketones are positive

■ your blood sugar has increased over the past 12 hours and the ketones are positive

■ you have nausea or vomiting

ASK YOUR DOCTOR OR DIABETES EDUCATOR ABOUT ADDING EXTRA RAPID-ACTING INSULIN WHEN THE KETONES ARE POSITIVE.

[1]These are guidelines, so please ask your doctor or diabetes educator for specific instructions.

These could mean KETO-ACIDOSIS—a DIABETIC EMERGENCY!

Acetest® tablets, Ketostix®, and Chemstrip K® are products for urine ketone testing that may be purchased at any pharmacy without a prescription. There is one meter called Precision Xtr which tests ketones in the blood. Contact your doctor or diabetes educator for information regarding this meter and ketone strips.

Helpful Hints for Urine Ketone Testing

- Be sure your timing is accurate—follow the instructions on the bottle.
- Keep the tablets or strips in a cool, dry place—out of sunlight. Do not leave them in a hot car.
- Buy one bottle at a time—remember to check the expiration date
- When comparing the colors of the tablets or strips to the chart, hold them close to the color chart.
- Good lighting is essential for obtaining accurate results.
- Do not store the tablets or strips in a bathroom—they can be ruined by moisture.

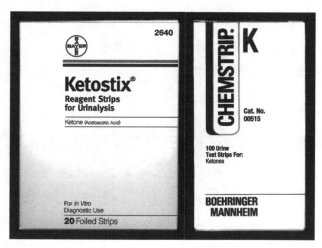

Medicines to Treat Diabetes

There are several different medicines used to treat diabetes. Each group of medicines works in a different way. You may be taking 1 or more of these medicines to control your blood sugar.

Following your meal plan and exercise program are very important in helping these medicines work.

Carry with you a list of all your medicines, including any other prescriptions, over-the-counter medicines, vitamins, minerals, and supplements. Write out the name, dose (example: number of milligrams, units, etc.), and when you take the medicines. Review the list with your doctor each visit.

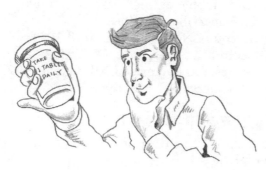

ORAL MEDICINES

Sulfonylureas			
Name	Tablet Size (mg)	Duration of Action (hr)	Maximum Dose (mg)
Dymelor/ Acetohexamide[a]	250 500	12–14	1,500
Diabinese/ Chlorpropamide[a]	100 250	36+	750
Tolinase/ Tolazamide[a]	100 250 500	12–24	1,000
Orinase/ Tolbutamide[a]	250 500	6–12	3,000
Micronase/Diabeta/ Glyburide[b,c]	1.25 2.5 5	24	20
Glucotrol/ Glipizide[d]	5 10	24	40
Glucotrol XL[e]/ Glipizide ER	2.5 5 10	24	20
Glynase/ Micronized Glyburide[f]	1.5 3 6	24	12
Amaryl/ Glimepiride[g]	1 2 4	24	8

[a]From *Diabetes Mellitus*, 8th edition, Lilly Research Laboratories, Indianapolis, IN, 1980.
[b]From Upjohn Therapeutic Profile of Micronase, May 1984.
[c]From Hoechst-Roussel, Somerville, NJ, 1984.
[d]From Roerig-Pfizer, Glucotrol, New York, NY, April 1994.
[e]From Pfizer-Pratt, Glucotrol XL, New York, NY, April 1994.
[f]From Upjohn, Glynase Prestabs, Kalamazoo, MI, March 1992.
[g]From Hoechst-Roussel, Somerville, NJ, December 1995.

■ Sulfonylureas help your pancreas make insulin.

■ These drugs are related to other sulfa drugs and can produce sulfa reactions, but they can be used with caution even when a known allergy to sulfa exists.

- They may be taken once or more than once a day.
- Side effects are usually minimal. They can include lack of appetite, nausea, vomiting, skin rash, headache, or hypoglycemia.
- To avoid low blood sugar (hypoglycemia) while taking these drugs, take only the prescribed amount of medication, and if meals are more than 4 or 5 hours apart, add a snack. Review pages 15–20 on hypoglycemia for treatment and prevention.
- *Caution:* If you drink alcohol while taking one of these drugs (particularly Diabinese/Chlorpropamide), you may have a reaction involving symptoms such as flushing; warm, tingling, burning sensations in the face and neck; and lightheadedness.
- Glucotrol or glipizide should be taken on an empty stomach ($\frac{1}{2}$ hour before your meal). Any of the other drugs may be taken just before the meal.
- If you forget to take a pill, take your usual dose the next time you are due to take one. DO NOT double the dose or try to "catch up" for the missed dose.
- When you must *fast* for blood work or a procedure, do not take your diabetes pill until you are ready to eat.

Meglitinides			
Name	Tablet size (mg)	Duration of Action (hr)	Maximum Dose (mg)
Prandin/ Repaglinide[a]	0.5 1 2	1.4	16
Starlix/ Nateglinide[b]	60 120	1.5	360

[a]From Novo Nordisk Pharmaceuticals, Inc., Princeton, NJ, 1997.
[b]From Novartis Pharmaceuticals Corporation, East Hanover, NJ, February 2001.

- When the blood sugar rises (after a meal), these pills help to control the rise by causing the pancreas to release more insulin. As the blood sugar lowers, the effects of the drugs decrease.

- They should be taken before a meal (0–30 minutes). If you miss a meal, you do not take the medication.

- Side effects are usually minimal. They can include hypoglycemia, nausea, headache, upset stomach, or diarrhea.

- If you forget to take your pill, take your usual dose the next time you are due to take it. DO NOT double the dose or try to "catch up" on missed doses.

Biguanides			
Name	Tablet Size (mg)	Duration of Action (hr)	Maximum Dose (mg)
Glucophage/ Metformin[a]	500 850 1,000	6	2,000
Glucophage XR/ Metformin ER[b]	500 750	6	2,000
Riomet/ liquid Metformin[c]	500mg/5mL	6	2,000
Fortamet/Metformin[d] (extended release)	500 1000	6	2,000
Glumetza/Metformin[e] (extended release)	500 1000	6	2,000

[a]From Bristol-Myers-Squibb, Princeton, NJ, February 1995.
[b]From Bristol-Myers-Squibb, Princeton, NJ, October 2000.
[c]From Ranbaxy Laboratories, Princeton, NJ, 2005.
[d]From Sciele Pharma Inc., Atlanta, GA, 2007.
[e]From Depomed, Inc., Menlo Park, CA, 2008.

- Glucophage lowers blood sugar mainly by working on the liver. It also helps glucose enter muscle and fat cells.

- When used alone, Glucophage does not cause low blood sugar (hypoglycemia).

- This drug will lower triglycerides, total cholesterol, and LDL (bad) cholesterol and increase HDL (good) cholesterol.

- It may help with weight loss.

- Side effects may include increased gas, nausea, cramping, feeling of fullness (bloating), diarrhea, and a metallic taste in the mouth. These symptoms will usually go away if Glucophage is started slowly, taken *with* food, and the dose is increased slowly.

- Glucophage XR or Metformin ER is given once a day and should be taken at the evening meal.

- Glucophage should be stopped before admission to the hospital or when having an x-ray or procedure involving dye. Discuss this with your doctor.

- Glucophage is not for everyone—only those who have good liver and kidney function can take it.

- You should not drink alcohol when taking Glucophage.

- If you forget your pill, take your usual dose the next time you are due to take it. DO NOT double the dose or try to "catch up" on missed doses.

Thiazolidinediones		
Name	*Tablet Size (mg)*	*Maximum Dose (mg)*
Avandia/Rosiglitazone[a]	2 4 8	8
Actos/Pioglitazone[b]	15 30 45	45

[a]From Smithkline Beecham Pharmaceuticals, Philadelphia, PA, May 1999.
[b]From Takeda Pharmaceuticals America, Inc., Lincolnshire, IL, July 1999.

- These drugs lower blood sugar by helping glucose and insulin enter muscle cells.

- They should be taken *with* the first meal of the day. If you forget it, take it with the next meal. Do not double the dose or try to "catch up" on missed doses.
- When used alone, they do not cause low blood sugar (hypoglycemia).
- If you are taking insulin or other diabetes pills, your dose may need to be lowered. Test your blood sugar, and your doctor will guide you.
- These drugs can interfere with some birth control pills—discuss this with your doctor.
- Because of the way these drugs work, it may take one to three months to see how well they will work for you.

Alpha-Glucosidase Inhibitors			
Name	*Tablet Size (mg)*	*Duration of Action (hr)*	*Maximum Dose (mg)*
Precose/ Acarbose[a]	25 50 100	2	300
Glyset/ Miglitol[b]	25 50 100	2	300

[a]From Bayer Pharmaceuticals Division, Wayne, NJ, 1997.
[b]From Pharmacia and Upjohn Company, New York, NY, 1999

- These drugs lower blood sugar by slowing the absorption of carbohydrates (starches or sugar) after a meal.
- They *must* be taken with the first bite of a meal, and the meal must include foods from the starch group (bread, rice, pasta, potatoes, cereal, beans, etc.).
- The most common side effects are diarrhea and increased gas. Starting with a low dose and raising the dose slowly will help limit these side effects.

- When used alone, they do not cause low blood sugar (hypoglycemia).

- Low blood sugar (hypoglycemia) can occur if these drugs are used with one of the sulfonylurea drugs (see pages 124–125) or insulin. Because of the way they work, the usual juices, soda, candy, and milk used to treat low blood sugar will not raise blood sugar—you must use glucose tablets or gels.

DPP-4 Inhibitor

Name	Tablet size (mg)		
Januvia/Sitagliptin[a]	25	50	100
Onglyza/Saxagliptin[b]	2.5	5	
Tradjenta/Linagliptin[c]	5		
Nesina/Alogliptin[d]	6.25	12.5	25

[a]From Merck & Co., Inc., Whitehouse Station, NJ, 2006.
[b]From Bristol-Myers Squibb, Princeton, NJ, 2009.
[c]From Boehringer Ingleheim Pharmaceuticals, Ridgefield, CT 06877, 2011
[d]From Takeda Pharmaceuticals America, Inc., Deerfield, IL 2013

- These medicines have several actions:
  1. lower blood sugar, especially after meals and between meals;
  2. improve the amount of insulin produced by your pancreas;
  3. decrease the amount of sugar made by the liver, especially at meal time.

- These medicines are not used to treat Type 1 diabetes.

- Possible side effects are: stuffy or runny nose, sore throat, cold, headache, nausea, or diarrhea.

- They may be taken with or without food.

SGLT2 Inhibitor		
Name	Tablet size (mg)	
Invokana/Canagliflozin[a]	100	300
Farxiga/Dapagliflozin[b]	5	10
Jardiance/Empagliflozin[c]	10	25

[a]From Janssen Pharmaceuticals, Inc., Titusville, NJ 08560 2013.
[b]From Bristol-Myers Squibb, Princeton, NJ, 2014.
[c]From Boehringer Ingleheim Pharmaceuticals, Ridgefield, CT, 2014.

- These medicines lower the blood sugar by causing the kidneys to throw away more glucose in the urine rather than putting as much glucose back into the blood.

- Take these medicines before the first meal of the day.

- You may have an increase in how often and how much you must urinate even at night.

- If you miss a dose, take it as soon as you remember it as long as it is not too close to the time the next dose is due.

- Side effects may include: dehydration (loss of body water and salt), which may make you feel dizzy, faint, lightheaded or weak especially when you stand up. You may be at greater risk for dehydration if you have low blood pressure, take medicines to lower your blood pressure, follow a low salt diet, have kidney problems, or are over 65 years of age.

   vaginal yeast infections

   yeast infections of the penis

   urinary tract infections

   high amount of potassium in your blood

- Hypoglycemia (low blood sugar, page 15–20) may occur if you are taking another diabetes medicine form the Sulfonylurea group (page 124–125) or an insulin (page 135–136).

Combination Medication

Name	Tablet size (mg)	Duration of Action	Maximum Dose (mg)
Glucovance[a] Glyburide and Metformin	1.25/250 2.5/500 5/500	24 hrs	10/2000 or 20/2000
Metaglip[b] Metformin and Glipizide	2.5/250 2.5/500 5/500	24 hrs	20/2000
Avandamet[c] Avandia and Metformin	1/500 2/500 4/500 2/1000 4/1000	24 hrs	8/2000
Actos plus Met[d] Actos and Metformin	15/500 15/850	24 hrs	45/2550
Avandaryl[e] Avandia and Glimpiride	4/1 4/2 4/4	24 hrs	8/8
Janumet[f] Januvia and Metformin	50/500 50/1000	24 hrs	100/2000
Prandimet[g] Prandin and Metformin	1/500 2/500	1.4–6	10/2500 in 24 hrs or 4/1000 per meal
Kombiglyze XR[h] Saxagliptin and Metformin	5/500 5/1000 2.5/1000	24 hrs	5/2000 in 24 hrs
Glyxambi[i]	10/5	24 hrs	25/5

[a]From Bristol-Myers Squibb Company, Princeton, NJ, August 2000.
[b]From Bristol-Myers Squibb Company, Princeton, NJ, October 2002.
[c]From GlaxoSmithKline, Research Triangle Park, NC, October 2002.
[d]From Takeda Pharmaceuticals, North America, Inc., 2005.
[e]From GlaxoSmithKline, Research Triangle Park, NC, December 2005.
[f]From Merck & Co., Whitehouse Station, NJ, 2007.
[g]From Novo Nordisk, Princeton, NJ 2008.
[h]From Bristol-Myers Squibb Co., Princeton, NJ, Nov. 2010.
[i]From Boehringer Ingelheim Pharmaceuticals,Inc., Ridgefield, CT
06877 and Eli Lilly & Company Indianapolis, IN 46285, 2015.

Combination Medicines (*continued*)

Name	Tablet size (mg)	Duration of Action	Maximum Dose (mg)
Jentadueto[j] Linagliptin and Metformin	2.5/500 2.5/850 2.5/1000	24 hrs	5/2000
Janumet XR[k] Janumet and Metformin extended release	100/1000 50/500 50/1000	24 hrs	100/2000
Kazano[l] Alogliptin and Metformin	12.5/500 12.5/1000	24 hrs	25/200
Oseni[m] Alogliptin and Pioglitizone	12.5/15 12.5/30 12.5/45 25/15 25/30 25/45	24 hrs	25/45
Invokamet[n] Invokana and Metformin	50/500 50/1000 150/500 150/1000	24 hrs	300/2000
Xigduo XR[o] Farxiga and Metformin XR	5/500 5/1000 10/500 10/1000	24 hrs	20/2000

[j]From Boehringer Ingelheim Pharmaceuticals, Inc., Ridgefort, CT, 2012
[k]From Merck and Company, Whitehouse Station, NY, 2012
[l,m]From Takeda Pharmaceuticals America, Inc., Deerfield, IL 2013.
[n]From Janssen Pharmaceuticals, Inc., Titusville, NJ 08560, 2014
[o]From AstraZeneca Pharmaceuticals LP, Wilmington, DE 19850, 2014

■ The above pills are all combinations of medications discussed earlier in this section. See pages 124–125 for information on Glyburide, Glipizide, and Glimepiride;

pages 126–127 for Metformin, pages 127–128 for Avandia and Actos; pages 125–126 for Prandin; page 129 for Januvia, Saxagliptin, Linagliptin, and Alogliptin; and page 130 for Farxiga, Invokana, and Jardiance.

There are certain other drugs that can affect the oral medications, so it is very important that you check with your doctor before taking any other medication and take only what your doctor prescribes.

Incretin Mimetic			
Name	Dose		
Byetta/Exenatide[a]	5 mcg	10 mcg	
Victoza/Liraglutide[b]	0.6 mg	1.2 mg	1.8 mg
Bydureon/exenatide extended release[c]	2 mg		
Tanzeum/Albiglutide[d]	30 mg 50	50 mg	10 mg
Trulicity /Dulaglutide[e]	.75 mg 1.5	1.5 mg	1.2 mg

[a]From Amylin Pharmaceuticals, Inc., San Diego, CA, and Eli Lilly and Company, Indianapolis, IN, 2005.
[b]From Novo Nordisk, Inc., Princeton, NJ, 2010.
[c]From Amylin Pharmaceuticals, Inc. , San Diego, CA 2012
[d]From GlaxoSmith Kline LLC, Wilmington, DE 19808, 2014
[e]From Eli Lilly and Company, Indianapolis, IN 46285, 2014

- These drugs have several actions; 1) help with producing insulin from the pancreas right after a meal; 2) stop the liver from producing too much sugar when it is not needed; 3) slow the rate in which food leaves the stomach; 4) help with weight loss.
- They work on the blood sugar rise after meals.
- They are given by injection (similar to insulin) with a prefilled pen. Byetta is given 5–60 minutes before the morning and evening meals. Victoza is given once a day.
- They are not used in Type 1 diabetes.
- Possible side effects include nausea, vomiting, diarrhea, feeling jittery, dizziness, headache, upset stomach, and low blood sugar.

- Medicines such as birth control pills and antibiotics should be taken 1 hour before the Byetta and Victoza.
- If you miss a dose, wait until the next time you are due to take them.
- Bydureon, Tanzeum and Trulicity are long acting and are given every 7 days at any time of the day.

Amylin Mimetic	
Name	Dose
Symlin[a]	30 µg (micrograms)
Pramlinitide acetate	60 µg
	90 µg
	120 µg

[a]From Amylin Pharmaceuticals, Inc., San Diego, CA, 2005.

- Amylin is used with insulin in Type 1 and Type 2 diabetes.
- It is given by injection the same way insulin is given.
- It is taken at the mealtime in addition to the usual dose of insulin. It cannot be mixed with insulin.
- Symlin has several actions: 1) it slows the rate in which food leaves the stomach; 2) it decreases the secretion of glucagon (a hormone that raises blood sugar); 3) it lowers blood sugars after meals; 4) it helps in losing weight.
- The storage of Symlin is the same as for insulin. See page 132.
- Side effects may include hypoglycemia, nausea, loss of appetite, vomiting, or diarrhea.

INSULIN

You may need insulin to keep your blood sugar in your acceptable range. People with Type 1 diabetes must take insulin every day. People with Type 2 diabetes may need insulin during times of stress such as illness, emotional trauma, pregnancy, infection, or when your own insulin cannot work well enough. Once the stressful event is over, it may be possible to stop taking insulin and control your blood sugar with diet or diet and an oral medicine.

If you are an overweight person with Type 2 diabetes taking insulin, weight loss (especially combined with exercise) will lower your blood sugar, and possibly allow you to stop the insulin.

Regardless of why you must take insulin, this section explains all you need to know and some "tricks of the trade" to make it easier.

From the tables on pages 135–136, choose your insulin(s) by its type and species and the company that makes it.

Lilly Insulin				
Type	Species	Onset (Hrs.)	Peak (Hrs.)	Duration (Hrs.)
I. Rapid-Acting				
A. Humalog[a]	Human	$1/4$	1–2	3–4
II. Short-Acting				
A. Humulin R	Human	$1/2$	2–4	6–8
III. Intermediate-Acting				
A. Humulin N	Human	1–2	6–12	18–24
IV. Mixtures				
A. Humulin 70/30	Human	$1/2$	6–12	18–24
B. Humalog Mix 75/25[b]	Human	$1/4$	2–12	22
C. Humalog Mix 50/50[c]	Human	$1/4$	2–12	22

[a] From Humalog®, Eli Lilly and Company, Indianapolis, IN, 1996.
[b] From Eli Lilly and Company, Indianapolis, IN, 2000.
[c] From Eli Lilly and Company, Indianapolis, IN, 2006.
Source: Insulin from Lilly, Eli Lilly and Company, Indianapolis, IN, 1994 and 1997.

Novo Nordisk				
Type	Species	Onset (Hrs.)	Peak (Hrs.)	Duration (Hrs.)
I. Rapid-Acting		10–20		
A. Novolog	Human	min.	1–3	3–5
II. Short-Acting				
A. Novolin R	Human	$1/_2$	$2^1/_2$–5	8
III. Intermediate-Acting				
A. Novolin N	Human	$1^1/_2$	4–12	24
IV. Long-Acting				
A. Levemir[a]	Human	5.7	no peak	24
V. Mixtures				
A. Novolin 70/30	Human	$1/_2$	4–12	24
B. NovologMix 70/30[b]	Human	$1/_4$	1–4	24

[a,b]Novo Nordisk Pharmaceuticals, Inc., Princeton, NJ, 2005.
Source: Novo Nordisk Pharmaceuticals, Princeton, NJ, 2004.

Sanofi				
Type	Species	Onset (Hrs.)	Peak (Hrs.)	Duration (Hrs.)
I. Rapid-Acting				
A. Apidra[a]	Human	$1/_4$	1–2	2–3
II. Long-Acting				
A. Lantus[b]	Human		no peak	24
B. Toujeo[c]	Human		no peak	24
	This is U-300, a stronger (concentrated) form of Lantus insulin.			

[a]Aventis Pharmaceuticals, Inc., Kansas City, MO, 2000.
[b]Aventis, 2004. [c]Aventis, 2015.

Inhaled Insulin				
Type	Species	Onset (Hrs.)	Peak (Hrs.)	Duration (Hrs.)
I. Afrezza[a]	Human	$1/_4$	1	3

[a]MannKind Corporation, Danbury, CT 06810, 2014

Regarding your insulin, it is VERY IMPORTANT for you to remember

- the name or type
- the species (human)
- the company that makes it
- the concentration (U-100)
- the dose (number of units)
- to check the expiration date

YOUR INSULIN INFORMATION TO REMEMBER:

Name _____

Species _____

Company _____

Concentration _____

Dose _____

Expiration date _____

Injection Time

When you inject your insulin depends on the type of insulin you are using. Some insulins are injected at mealtimes and others can be taken at bedtime. Ask your doctor or diabetes educator when you should take your insulin.

Insulin Storage

Insulin comes in bottles (called vials) or pens. The best place to store your insulin is in the refrigerator on the door (whether opened or not). Once the insulin vial or pen is opened for use, it may be stored at room temperature (40°–86° F) for 14(pen)–28(vial) days. Check the directions that come in the box with the insulin for the exact number of days. Write the date on the insulin vial or pen when you open it.

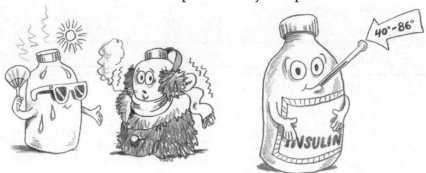

Protect insulin from sunlight and do not let it freeze. Do not store it in places such as cars, bathrooms, or kitchens. Even if it is stored in the refrigerator, you should throw away any vial/pen of insulin that has been open for more than 14 days for the pen and 28 days for the vial. The insulin begins to lose its ability to work correctly.

Hint: If you inject room-temperature insulin instead of cold insulin, you can avoid any stinging feeling and get better absorption into your tissues.

THE INSULIN SYRINGE

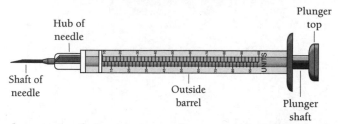

The only parts of the syringe that you should touch are the parts that do not enter the body or come into contact with the insulin. You can touch

- the needle hub
- the outside of the barrel
- the plunger top

If you touch parts of the syringe that enter your body during an injection, you will make the syringe dirty and run the risk of giving yourself an infection. You should never touch

- the shaft of the needle
- the inside of the barrel

Reusing Insulin Syringes

Many people reuse their insulin syringes, and researchers are now reporting that this practice is okay for most diabetics. (Suggested use is 1–2 times per syringe.) You must be very careful when drawing up the insulin and giving yourself the injection to keep the syringe and needle very clean. Check with your doctor or diabetes educator as to whether or not you should reuse your insulin syringes.

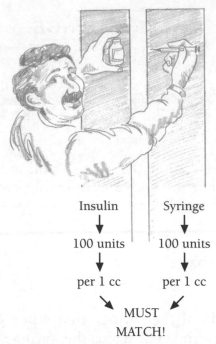

Insulin   Syringe
↓   ↓
100 units   100 units
↓   ↓
per 1 cc   per 1 cc
↘   MUST   ↙
         MATCH!

Be sure to buy the proper syringe for the strength of insulin you are taking! If you have the wrong syringe, you will not be giving yourself the right amount of insulin. You will probably be taking U-100 insulin, because this is the most common insulin made in the United States. (U-40 and U-80 insulins are no longer made in the United States.) "U-100" means that there are 100 units of insulin in 1 cc.

INJECTION TECHNIQUE

Using One Type of Insulin

Outlined below are steps to guide you in preparing your insulin for injection.

1. Wash your hands.
2. Gather your equipment: insulin, syringe, alcohol.

3. ROLL (20 times) the insulin bottle between your hands—make sure the insulin is well mixed.

4. Cleanse the top of the insulin bottle with the alcohol and let it dry.

5. Put the needle into the bottle of insulin. Keeping the needle in the bottle, turn it completely upside down. Pull down the plunger quickly to fill the syringe with more insulin than you need (about 10 units over your dose).

6. Push it all back into the bottle and repeat step 5.

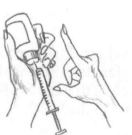

7. Now measure the amount of insulin you need by sliding the plunger back up to the correct marking.

8. Check the syringe for air bubbles, because they take the place of insulin in the syringe and will prevent you from getting the proper amount. If you see any bubbles, repeat steps 6 and 7.

9. Once a week, remove the plunger from the syringe and put the needle into the bottle for 2 to 3 seconds. This will keep the air pressure inside the insulin bottle equal to the pressure outside of it.

Throughout the process of drawing the insulin and giving the injection, be very careful not to touch the needle or lay it down. If you do get the needle dirty, throw away the syringe and start again with a new one.

A shortened version of drawing a single insulin:

1. Roll insulin bottle (20 times), cleanse top.
2. Put needle into bottle of insulin.
3. Turn bottle upside down.
4. Pull down quickly—beyond what you need.
5. Push all of the insulin back into the bottle.
6. Pull down quickly again—beyond what you need.
7. Measure exact amount of insulin needed.
8. Check for air bubbles.

Using Two Types of Insulin

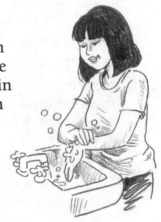

Listed below are steps to guide you in mixing two types of insulin in one syringe for injection. (Cloudy insulin refers to NPH insulin, and clear insulin refers to Regular, Novolog, Humalog, or Apidra).

1. Wash your hands.
2. Gather your equipment: insulins, syringe, and alcohol.
3. ROLL (20 times) the insulin bottles between your hands—make sure the insulin is well mixed.

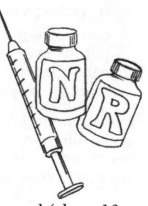

4. Cleanse the tops of the insulin bottles with alcohol and let them dry.
5. Put the needle into the bottle of clear insulin and turn it completely upside down. Pull the plunger down quickly to fill the syringe with more insulin than you need (about 10 units more).

6. Push it all back into the bottle, and repeat the last step.

7. Now measure the exact amount of clear insulin you need.

8. Check for air bubbles, because they take the place of insulin in the syringe and will prevent you from getting the proper amount. If you see any bubbles, repeat steps 6 and 7.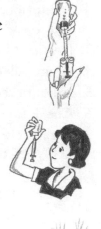

9. Now put your needle into the cloudy insulin bottle and SLOWLY draw the amount of cloudy insulin you need. Remember, you already have clear insulin in your syringe, so the total amount of insulin in your syringe should equal the TOTAL of both the clear and cloudy insulins.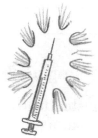

Throughout the process of drawing the insulin and giving the injection, be very careful not to touch the needle or lay it down. If you do get the needle dirty, throw away the syringe and start again with a new one.

A shortened version of mixing two insulins:

1. Roll bottles (20 times) , cleanse tops.
2. Put needle into the clear insulin—keep needle in bottle and turn upside down. Draw out quickly—beyond what you need.
3. Push all of it back into the bottle.
4. Again, pull down quickly—beyond what you need.
5. Measure the exact amount of clear insulin you need.
6. Check for air bubbles.
7. Put needle into the cloudy insulin and draw down SLOWLY to the TOTAL amount you need.

_____ units of clear insulin (Regular, Humalog, Novolog, or Apidra)

_____ units of cloudy insulin (NPH)

_____ TOTAL amount of insulin to inject

Using an Insulin Pen

Listed below are the steps to guide you in preparing your insulin pen for the injection.

1. Wash your hands.
2. Gather your equipment—pen and pen needle.
3. If the insulin is a cloudy one, roll and turn the pen several times to mix the insulin evenly in the pen.
4. Attach the pen needle to the pen and remove the caps—there are two.
5. Measure 1–2 units of insulin and push out (waste) the insulin. Be sure you see a drop of insulin at the end of the pen needle. The directions with the insulin pens call this an airshot or safety shot.
6. Now measure the dose of insulin that you need.

Giving Your Injection

Now you are ready to give your injection. These steps are outlined to guide you.

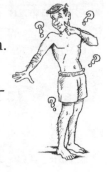

1. Choose a site for the injection—if necessary, cleanse it with soap and water. If you use alcohol, let the skin dry before injecting the insulin.

2. Pinch the skin between your thumb and fingers.

3. Quickly insert the syringe or insulin pen at either a 90-degree or a 60-degree angle to the skin. Your diabetes educator will guide you as to the angle.

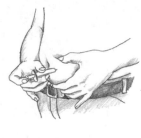

4. Inject the insulin.

5. Count 2 seconds if using a syringe or 5–10 seconds if using an insulin pen and then pull out the needle.

DON'T DISPOSE OF SYRINGES/PEN NEEDLES CARELESSLY. Before we move on to another section we would like to think about how to throw away your used syringes/pen needles known as "sharps."

As the result of a new law in 2008, you can no longer throw your syringes/pen needles in the garbage. Check with your city or local garbage/trash company for directions on how to throw away these "sharps." Most cities/trash companies are setting up special programs.

Safely throw away your sharps by:

- getting an approved sharps (red) container from your city or trash company or local pharmacy

- fill it about 3/4 full—not completely full

- store your sharps container in an area that is safe from children and animals.

- check your city's hazardous waste collection dates or local fire departments for throwing away your sharps containers.

Areas of Injection

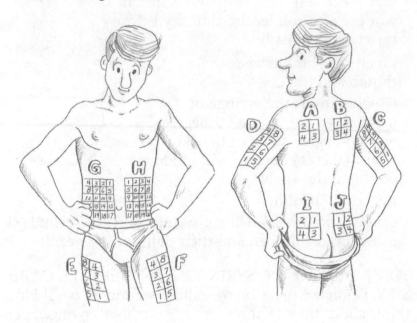

The pictures above show you the areas of the body that are best for insulin injection because they are away from joints, nerves, and large blood vessels.

There are three ways to rotate your injection sites. One way is to use all injection sites in one area (for example 1–8 in boxes C and D) before moving to the next area. The second way is to use just the abdomen and make use all the sites you have in that one area. The third way is to choose specific areas for certain types of insulin or times of the day. Ask your doctor or diabetes educator for guidance.

You may need to change your pattern when you plan to exercise. Insulin injected near a muscle to be used in exercise will be more rapidly absorbed because of the increased blood flow. This gives you a greater chance of having hypoglycemia, so, on occasion, you may need to change your injection pattern and use an area away from the muscles you plan to use during exercise.

> It is important to ROTATE YOUR SITES so that you do not develop an abscess or infection or a hardened area at an injection site. Give your injections $^1/_2$ inch apart (the width of your finger). The U-100 insulins are purer than the older insulins, and they are less likely to cause skin problems from long-term use.

We strongly recommend that a family member or close friend know how to give you insulin injections. There may be a time when you are too ill to give yourself your injection, or you just may want a day off once in a while. Maybe others can reach sites you are unable to reach. Your arm is the most difficult place in which to give yourself a proper injection, so let others use this site. For children, the sites located on the buttocks and shoulders are good ones for parents and others to use.

Insulin Pumps

Another way to give insulin is through an insulin pump. The pumps are battery operated, are the size of a pager, and weigh a few ounces. A rapid-acting insulin is delivered to the body through a thin plastic tubing into a needle inserted under the skin in the abdomen (the needle is changed every 2 days). A steady amount of insulin (called basal insulin) is given continuously, and then additional doses of insulin (called boluses) are given at mealtimes. The blood sugar is tested frequently throughout the day, and the pump is adjusted to deliver the amount of insulin that the body needs.

Wearing an insulin pump can provide better blood sugar control because of the constant infusion of insulin, the careful monitoring of the blood sugar, and the frequent adjustment of insulin doses.

If you would like more information about insulin pumps, please talk with your doctor or diabetes educator, or check these websites:

Medtronicdiabetes.com

Animas.com

Accu-chekinsulinpump.com

Myomnipod.com

Tandemdiabetes.com

Snapppump.com

There are glucose monitoring systems that monitor your blood sugar over 24 hour periods of time. These "continuous glucose monitors" are often used with insulin pumps. Check these websites for more information:

DexCom.com

Medtronicdiabetes.com

Abbottdiabetes.com

REMEMBER: All these medicines help to control your blood sugar; they cannot do it alone, nor can they *cure* diabetes. The MEDICINES need YOUR HELP to work.

Follow your meal plan.   Exercise.   Test your blood sugar.

Laboratory Tests

FASTING BLOOD SUGAR

This test measures the amount of sugar in your blood after you have fasted for 8–12 hours. A normal fasting blood sugar result is under 100 milligrams. See page 28 for the acceptable range for those who have diabetes.

When you are to have a fasting blood sugar, do not eat or drink after midnight the night before until after a blood sample is drawn in the morning (small sips of water are allowed).

If you have diabetes, do not take your diabetes medicine until after the blood is drawn *and you are ready to eat*.

POST-PRANDIAL BLOOD SUGAR

This test measures the amount of sugar in your blood 2 hours after you eat a normal meal. When your doctor orders this test, you should

1. Take your diabetes medicine as usual.
2. Eat your normal meal at your usual time.

3. Test your blood sugar 2 hours later—2 hours after the start of the meal.

If your blood sugar is too high, it may mean that changes are needed in your meal plan, insulin, or oral medication. If your blood sugar is under good control, the result should be in the acceptable range (under 180).

REMEMBER: A one-time fasting or post-prandial blood sugar test may not reflect your TOTAL control—these tests are only used as guidelines for you and your doctor.

ESTIMATED AVERAGE GLUCOSE (eAG)

(formerly known as Hemoglobin A1c)

Sugar attaches to hemoglobin (red blood cells) and remains there for the life time of the cells which is 120 days.

The result of this blood test, Hemoglobin A1c, tells you and your doctor how well your blood sugars have been controlled over the last 2–3 months. Think of it as an average of all your blood sugars for every moment of every day for that period of time.

Here is a chart to help you see the result of the Hemoglobin A1c (in a percentage %) and what it means as your average blood glucose.

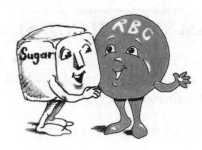

Hemoglobin A1c *Result in %*	*estimated Average Glucose* *eAG in mg/dl*	
5	97	
5.5	111	Normal
6	126	
6.5	140	GOAL
7	154	
7.5	169	
8	183	
8.5	197	
9	212	
9.5	226	
10	240	Too high
10.5	255	
11	269	
11.5	283	
12	298	
12.5	312	
13	326	

The Hemoglobin A1c test should be done every 3–6 months so that you have a lab result giving you a measure of your estimated Average Glucose (eAG) to compare with your averages of the blood sugars taken with your meter.

If you test your blood sugar before and 2 hours after different meals, you should find your glucose meter results close to your lab result of estimated Average Glucose (eAG). You are checking your blood sugar at times when it is lower such as before meals and at times when it is higher such as after meals.

If you test your blood sugar only in the morning or before meals, you may find your glucose meter results are lower than your lab result of estimated Average Glucose (eAG). This is because you are testing when the blood sugar tends to be lower and are missing the spike in your blood sugar after meals.

A normal Hemoglobin A1c is less than 5.7%.

When you have diabetes or prediabetes, your GOAL is:

Estimated Average Glucose (eAG)   Under 140–145*

Hemoglobin A1c   6.5%–7%*

*But these goals may need to be adjusted for you with your
  health care provider.

CHAPTER 10

Exercise

Exercise has been proven to be EXTREMELY important in the control of blood sugar. In fact, for the majority of people with Type 2 diabetes, exercise in combination with weight loss is all that is needed to control their blood sugar.

During exercise, body cells are much more sensitive to insulin and glucose, allowing the body to burn the glucose for energy while requiring a smaller amount of insulin—it works on the "insulin resistance" (see page 3).

THE BENEFITS

There are many benefits of exercise:

It helps you lose weight.

It is helpful in maintaining your weight.

It is helpful in decreasing the amount of medication (insulin and oral medication) you must take.

It can reduce your blood sugar.

It reduces your blood pressure.

It reduces your resting heart rate.

It strengthens your heart.

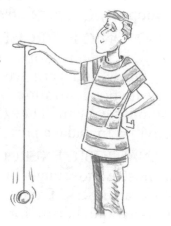

It raises your HDL (good) cholesterol.

It increases blood circulation.

It increases your energy.

It reduces the effects of stress on your body.

It helps your lungs work better, making breathing easier.

It makes you feel better about yourself.

All these benefits from exercise translate into a "physically fit" body, that is, a body whose heart, lungs, and muscles can work better for you with less effort.

THE TYPES

There are different types of exercises that do different things for your body. Let's take a look at what they are.

ISOMETRIC EXERCISES contract muscles without producing movement. In other words, they tense muscles against other muscles or objects that do not move. Some muscles are strengthened, but they produce tension within the muscles, causing a rise in blood pressure. For this reason, people with high blood pressure, heart problems, or diabetic retinopathy (see page 189) should avoid these exercises.

ISOTONIC EXERCISES tone muscles and burn calories. They are usually stop-and-start activities such as calisthenics, house and yard work, bowling, and golfing. Because they are not continuous activities, they cannot, alone, make you physically fit. They (calisthenics in particular) are good activities to make a *part* of your complete exercise program.

ANAEROBIC EXERCISES are exercises that involve a lot of muscle movement but never last long enough to affect physical fitness. Examples include walking five flights of stairs, a quick run for the bus, the 100-yard dash, and swimming sprints. Doing these occasionally will not help you develop physical fitness.

AEROBIC EXERCISES are continuous activities that use major muscle groups and last long enough to utilize oxygen and raise the heart rate to levels that develop and maintain physical fitness. Some examples are walking, jogging, swimming, biking, stationary biking, exercising on treadmills or rowing machines, and jumping rope. This is the type of exercise you must do to achieve all the benefits listed on pages 153–154, and to make your body physically fit.

The best program of exercise combines isotonic and aerobic exercise. When planning the aerobic part, you may choose more than one activity. One day you may enjoy walking, and the next you might try swimming. Changing activities helps you use different muscles.

THE PARTS OF AN EXERCISE PROGRAM

A complete program of exercise includes 4 parts:

1. Warm-up   3. Training or aerobic exercise

2. Stretching   4. Cool-down

Warm-up The warm-up session is 5 minutes of walking or a "slowed-down" version of the aerobic activity you plan to do. This allows you to slowly build up your heart rate and the blood flow to your muscles.

Stretching Allow 5–10 minutes for stretching exercises to loosen your muscles and joints and prevent muscle soreness and injury.

Stretch all the muscles in your body—neck, shoulders, back, arms, abdomen, hips, legs, ankles, and feet. Be careful not to bounce during your stretching or stretch to the point of feeling pain.

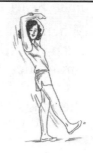

Training or aerobic exercise This is the main part of your exercise program, where you strengthen your heart and lungs and move your body toward physical fitness. At first you may only be able to do your activity of choice for 1–5 minutes, but you should *gradually* increase your exercise over time to 20–30 minutes of continuous activity.

Cool-down The cool-down session is actually a combination of the warm-up and stretching periods. Do your aerobic activity at a slow pace for about 5 minutes, and then do stretching exercises for another 5 minutes. This allows your heart rate and circulation to slow down.

What aerobic activity do you plan to do?

HOW HARD TO EXERCISE

Your heart rate is the measure of how hard your heart is working. To get the most benefit from your exercise, your heart rate must reach and maintain (for 20–30 minutes) a certain number of beats per minute during the training or aerobic exercise. This is known as your TARGET HEART RATE.

How do you determine your target heart rate? Follow these steps:

1. Subtract your age from 220 to determine your *maximum* heart rate.

2. When first starting an exercise program, it is better to keep your heart rate between 60 and 75% of your maximum heart rate. Multiplying your maximum heart rate by 0.6 (60%), and then by 0.75 (75%), gives you the range of your target heart rate.

3. After you have been exercising for a while, you will want to keep your heart rate between 75 and 85% of your maximum heart rate. Multiply your maximum heart rate by 0.75 (75%), and then by 0.85 (85%), to get the range of your target heart rate.

An easy way to measure your heart rate is to count the number of beats in 6 seconds, then add a zero. This gives you an estimate of your heart rate per minute.

Example #1 John is 55 years old and wants to be sure he is reaching and maintaining his target heart rate during the training or aerobic part of his exercise. To figure his target heart rate, take

$$\begin{array}{r} 220 \\ \underline{-\ 55}\ \text{(John's age)} \\ =\ 165\ \text{(John's maximum heart rate)} \end{array}$$

0.6 × 165 = 99 (60% of John's maximum heart rate)

0.75 × 165 = 124 (75% of John's maximum heart rate)

Because John is just beginning his exercise program, it is best for him to keep his heart rate between 99 and 124 (60–75% of his maximum heart rate).

Example #2 Jean is 65 years old and for the last 12 months has been walking for exercise. She wants to be certain she is reaching and maintaining her target heart rate during exercise. To figure Jean's target heart rate, take

$$\begin{array}{r} 220 \\ \underline{-\ 65}\ \text{(Jean's age)} \\ =\ 155\ \text{(Jean's maximum heart rate)} \end{array}$$

0.75 × 155 = 116 (75% of Jean's maximum heart rate)

0.85 × 155 = 132 (85% of Jean's maximum heart rate)

Because Jean has been exercising for a while, she should keep her heart rate between 116 and 132 (75–85% of her maximum heart rate).

Figure out your own target heart rate, or use this chart as a guideline.

	Beats per Minute		
Age	*60%*	*75%*	*85%*
20	120	150	170
25	117	146	166
30	114	142	161
35	111	138	157
40	108	135	153
45	105	131	148
50	102	127	144
55	99	123	140
60	96	120	136
65	93	116	131
70	90	112	127
75	87	108	123
80	84	105	119

For the 3 levels, my target heart rates are

60% _____

75% _____

85% _____

CAUTION: DISCUSS YOUR TARGET HEART RATE WITH YOUR DOCTOR. Some of you may be taking medications that do not allow your heart rate to increase during exercise, and therefore this information does not work for you. You will need special instruction.

During the training or aerobic part of your exercise take your pulse to determine whether you are exercising at your target heart rate. Check the rate about 3 minutes into your exercise, then count your pulse again a little over halfway through.

If your pulse rate is within your target heart rate	➜	you are working your heart and lungs just right.
If your pulse rate is above your target heart rate	➜	you are working too hard, so slow down a little.
If your pulse rate is below your target heart rate	➜	you are not working enough, so speed up a little.

How to Take Your Pulse

When taking your pulse, you will need a clock or watch with a second hand.

1. Take the first 2 fingers of one hand and place them on the wrist bone on the thumb side of your other hand.

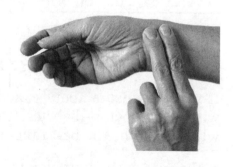

2. Move your fingers about one-quarter inch toward the underside of your wrist.

3. When you feel the heart beat (your pulse), count the number of beats for 6 seconds.

4. Add a zero to the number. This is your heart rate per minute.

If you do not want to measure your pulse, a simple way to judge your exercise is:

Not working enough   ➜   can sing while exercising

Working enough   ➜   can talk, but a little out of breath

Working too hard   ➜   too out of breath to talk

HOW OFTEN TO EXERCISE

BE CONSISTENT, and exercise a minimum of four or five times per week. Exercise at least every other day. Do not exercise 3 days in a row and then stop for the next four.

- If you are exercising to lose weight, you should exercise 5 or 6 times per week.
- Exercising every other day allows time for your muscles to rest.

What days do you plan to exercise?

WHEN TO EXERCISE

If you are unsure about exactly when to exercise, discuss with your doctor, diabetes educator, or exercise specialist what would be the best time of day for you.

- Exercise when your blood sugar tends to be the highest— 1 to 2 hours after a meal, or exercise in the morning *before* you take your diabetes medicine and eat breakfast.
- If it is best for you to exercise just before a meal, ask

your doctor or diabetes educator if you need to make any food and/or medication adjustments.

What time of the day is best for you to exercise?

WHEN NOT TO EXERCISE

■ If you have Type 1 diabetes and your blood sugar before exercise is over 250, skip the exercise session—it may raise your blood sugar even more.

■ If you have Type 1 diabetes, check your urine for ketones before you exercise. If they are negative (no ketones in the urine), go ahead and exercise. If there are ketones in the urine, do not exercise.

■ Do not exercise when you are ill.

WARNING SIGNS TO STOP EXERCISE

If you feel any of these symptoms during exercise, stop and rest.

■ Chest pain or pressure
■ Feeling dizzy or faint
■ Feeling unusually tired
■ Irregular heartbeat
■ Excessive sweating
■ Difficulty breathing

If the symptoms last longer than 5 minutes after you have stopped your exercise, seek medical help right away.

GUIDELINES FOR EXERCISING

- Choose an activity you will enjoy.

- **DISCUSS YOUR PLANS FOR EXERCISE WITH YOUR DOCTOR OR DIABETES EDUCATOR BEFORE STARTING YOUR PROGRAM.**

  This is true for all those who have diabetes, but especially for those who have any of the complications of diabetes (see pages 187–192) or any other health problems.

- It is wise to avoid activities that require a group of people, since you will be dependent on too many people for your exercise. It is also wise not to exercise alone. Choose one person to be your exercise partner, then you can encourage and support each other.

- When you are just beginning, you may be able to exercise at a training or aerobic level for only a few minutes at a time. Be patient and build your time gradually to 20–30 minutes of aerobic exercise per session.

- Have a thorough knowledge of hypoglycemia, as well as how to treat or prevent a reaction. BE PREPARED! *Always* carry a fast sugar food with you.

- Always have diabetic identification on your person (see page 173–174).

- Keep checking your blood sugar—this will give you information about food or medication adjustments that may be necessary, whether or not you should exercise on a particular day, and how exercise affects your blood sugar.

- Discuss with your doctor or diabetes educator YOUR NEEDS for medication and/or food adjustments before, during, or after exercise.

- Wait 1 hour after eating a meal before exercising, to allow time for your food to be digested.

- If you take insulin, inject it into an area that will not be used during the exercise (see page 146). If the insulin is injected into an area that will be exercised, it will be absorbed more rapidly and, possibly, cause low blood sugar. For example, if you are going to walk or run, you should inject the insulin into your arm or abdomen and not into a site on your leg.

- Drink plenty of fluids before, during, and after exercising.

- Pay attention to your feet—wear properly fitting, comfortable shoes. Check your feet daily for sores, blisters, and calluses.

REMEMBER: EXERCISE IS TREATMENT. The more you exercise the less medication you will need.

SOURCES OF INFORMATION ON EXERCISE

Aerobics for Women, by Mildred Cooper and Kenneth Cooper, M.D., M.P.H. Bantam Books, New York, 1972.

The Aerobics Program for Total Well-Being: Exercise, Diet, & Emotional Balance, by Kenneth Cooper, M.D., M.P.H. Bantam Books, New York, 1982.

Armchair Fitness: Aerobics, a video with three 20-minute routines of stretching and strengthening motions with music for anyone able to sit in a chair. Available from the Joslin Diabetes Center, Boston.

Chair Dancing Videos, by Jodi Stolove. Available from Chair Dancing International, Inc., 2658 Del Mar Heights Road, Del Mar, CA 92014. Call (800)551-4FUN or Fax (858)793-0747 or www.chairdancing.com.

Diabetes Sports and Exercise Book, by Claudia Graham, Ph.D., C.D.E.; Barbara Toohey; and June Biermann. Lowell House, Los Angeles, 1995.

Diabetes: Your Complete Exercise Guide, by Neil F. Gordon, M.D., Ph.D. Human Kinetics Publishers, Champaign, IL, 1993.

The Fitness Book for People with Diabetes, by W. Guyton Hornsby, Jr., Ph.D., C.D.E., 1994. Susan H. Lau, American Diabetes Association, Alexandria, VA.

The Ultimate Fit or Fat, by Covert Bailey, Houghton Mifflin Co., New York, 1999.

The Diabetic Athlete, by Sheri Colberg, Ph.D. 2001.

CHAPTER 11

Sick Days

Colds, flu, infections, injuries, surgery, and stressful times raise your blood sugar levels and may increase your need for insulin. When your blood sugar goes up, it is time to put into action your sick day plan. BEFORE the need arises, work out YOUR sick day plan with your doctor or diabetes educator so you will BE PREPARED!

If you do not yet have a sick day plan, follow these suggestions:

- NEVER omit your daily dose of insulin or oral medication. Take your usual dose.
- Test your blood sugar at least 2–4 times a day (before each meal and at bedtime)—sometimes you will need to test every 2 hours.
- If you have Type 1 diabetes, test your urine for ketones at least 4 times a day.
- Call your doctor for help

    If your blood sugar is difficult to control or greater than 300 mg

    If you are vomiting or have severe diarrhea or a fever

    If the illness lasts longer than 72 hours with no improvement

    If your urine tests positive for ketones

- Conserve your energy—REST!

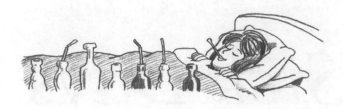

■ Drink large amounts of water and sugar-free liquids. Some examples are Propel, decaffeinated tea, sugar-free soda, sugar-free juices, sugar-free Snapple, and sugar-free carbonated waters. If you are unable to eat your usual meal, try to take the carbohydrate parts of your diet in liquids or semi-liquids—regular carbonated soft drinks,[1] broths (use sodium free if you have a restriction), fruits, fruit juices, Jell-O, and so on. You should take about 10–20 grams of carbohydrate every 1–2 hours while you are awake. Check your milk, bread, and fruit choice lists for the food, amount, and carbohydrate content.

Fruit: 1 serving = 15 grams carbohydrate

Milk: 1 serving = 12 grams carbohydrate

Bread: 1 serving = 15 grams carbohydrate

■ Return to your normal eating pattern as soon as possible.

When you are sick you may wish to take medicines to help ease your symptoms. There are many over-the-counter (nonprescription) medicines to help you, but be careful when choosing them. Check what is in the medicine—

---

[1]If blood tests are high for sugar, use sugar-free drinks instead of sweetened drinks.

sugar, alcohol, dextrose, and so on. Some medicines do affect your blood sugar, blood pressure, so ask your pharmacist for help in choosing the right one.

Carbohydrate Content of Common Foods

Amount	Food	Grams of Carbohydrate
½ cup	regular soft drinks (7-Up, cola, ginger ale), *not diet*	10
⅓ cup	regular Jell-O	15
½ cup	apple or pineapple juice	15
⅓ cup	grape or prune juice	15
½ cup	orange or grapefruit juice	15
½ cup	vanilla ice cream	15
¼ cup	sherbet	15
½ cup	frozen yogurt	15
1 slice	toast	15
6	saltine crackers	15
7	Ritz crackers	15
3 2½ inch squares	graham crackers	15
½ twin	Popsicle, regular	10
¾ cup	regular Gatorade	15
½ cup	cooked cereal	15
½ cup	custard or regular pudding	15
⅓ cup	tapioca	15
2 cups	broth-based soup, mixed with water	15

Carbohydrate Content of Common Foods (*cont.*)		
1 cup	creamed soup	15
1 cup	plain or sugar-free yogurt	12
1 tablespoon	Coke syrup	10
½ cup	sugar-free pudding	15

MY SICK DAY PLAN:

How often should I test my blood sugar when I am ill?

_____

Do I need to test my urine for ketones?

_____

If yes, how often?

_____

When should I call my doctor?

_____

Who will help me manage my blood sugar when I am ill?

_____

Who will help me manage my medications when I am ill?

_____

Who will help me manage my food and liquids when I am ill?

_____

Medication plan (how to adjust my insulin or oral medication) for illness:

_____

_____

_____

CHAPTER 12

Personal Hygiene

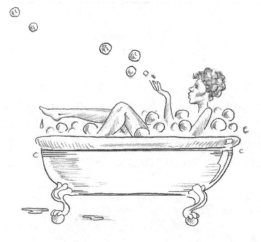

Your skin is the body's first line of defense against infection. It is very important to keep it clean, as well as protect it against cracks, cuts, sores, and so on, because infections can play havoc with your ability to control your blood sugars.

When blood sugars are poorly controlled, diabetes can cause a decrease in the blood supply to the legs and feet, leading to poor healing. If you smoke, the nicotine in cigarettes can damage blood vessels, also causing a decrease in blood flow to the legs and feet.

Poorly controlled blood sugar can damage nerves, resulting in a loss of feeling. When the legs or feet are numb, you are unable to feel pain when your feet are injured. Poor blood supply and lack of feeling make it quite easy for a small problem to turn into a serious problem quickly.

> The first step in preventing foot problems is to gain good control of your blood sugar. The second step is having good foot-care habits to prevent injury to your feet. And, finally, SEEK MEDICAL HELP IMMEDIATELY for any problems such as cuts or blisters that are not healing, corns, and calluses.

SKIN CARE

Bacteria, yeast, and fungus are found on the skin of all people. They tend to set up housekeeping and form skin infections in areas of the body that are dark, moist, and warm. This includes the vaginal and groin area, under the arms, and under the crease of the breasts.

> Notify your doctor if you
> - Have unusual itching
> - Notice a foul odor or discharge
> - Notice a rash
> - Notice a cut or bruise that is not healing
>
> Remember, skin infections can be both bothersome and dangerous. If found early, they can be treated easily, and you can prevent them with good blood sugar control.
>
> Again, DO NOT USE home remedies.

FOOT CARE

Here is a list of some DO's and DON'Ts of foot care:

Do's

- LOOK AT ALL AREAS of your feet and legs daily. Use a mirror if necessary to see all areas of your feet.

- Dry thoroughly, especially between the toes, with a soft towel.

- Apply lotion to soften the skin— but not between your toes.

- Wash your feet in warm water with mild soap.

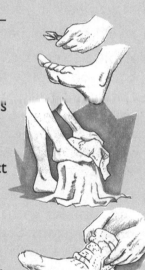

- Clip your toenails straight across the tops, and file the edges so there are no sharp points.

- Wear shoes at all times to protect your feet. Bedroom slippers should not be worn all day.

- Be sure your shoes are comfortable and fit properly.

- Change your socks or nylons daily.

- Break in new shoes slowly—wear them only 30 minutes the first day, and increase your wearing time by one-half hour each day.

- Ingrown toenails, corns, calluses, and so on should be treated by your doctor or a podiatrist (a foot specialist).

- Foot powder (used sparingly) can help reduce dampness caused by sweating feet.

- 24–48 hour rule—If anything on your feet is not healing well within 24–48 hours, seek medical help. Do not delay in getting quick and proper treatment for anything unusual on your feet.

- Check inside your shoes with your hand to make sure there are no stones, sharp objects, folded insoles, or anything else that could injure your feet.

Don'ts

- Never walk in your bare feet.

- Avoid socks and nylons that cause blisters.

- Avoid extremes of heat and cold—do not use hot water bottles, ice packs, or heating pads on your feet. Do not test water temperature with your feet—use your elbow.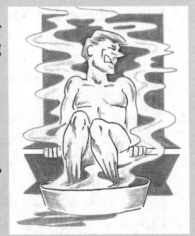

- Do not attempt home remedies for corns, calluses, or other sores. See your doctor or a podiatrist.

- Avoid garters or any other restrictive clothing on your feet and legs.

- Avoid crossing your legs.

- Do not routinely soak your feet unless it is approved by your doctor or podiatrist.

- Do not smoke—it cuts down the blood flow to your legs and feet.

REMEMBER: AVOID HOME REMEDIES—see your doctor immediately for treatment.

CHAPTER 13

Medical Identification

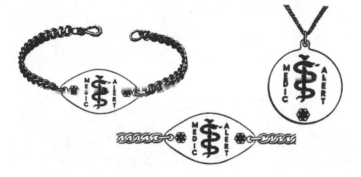

It is of utmost importance that you have some type of
diabetic identification ON YOUR PERSON at all times.

There are various ways of obtaining such an ID. You can get
one through your local chapter of the American Diabetes
Association (their phone number is in the telephone book).
Many pharmacies and jewelry stores carry various forms of
medical identification bracelets and necklaces. Through the
Medic Alert Foundation you can obtain an ID that includes
allergies or medical problems in addition to the diabetes.

Their address and phone number are 2323 Colorado Avenue, Turlock, CA 95382, (888)633-4298, or website is www.med-icalert.org, fax (209)669-2450. You can get an application at most pharmacies, hospitals, and chapters of the American Diabetes Association, or by writing directly to the Medic Alert Foundation.

CHAPTER 14

Stress

Stress affects everyone. It can be physical (such as pain, dehydration, fever, illness, accident, or hypoglycemia) or emotional (such as anger, fear, or worry).

Some stress is normal, but prolonged stress can lead to hyperglycemia (high blood sugar).

During a stressful situation there are certain "stress" hormones produced in a person's body. These hormones are adrenalin, glucagon, growth hormone, and cortisol. They work to raise the blood sugar in response to the stressful situation. This extra glucose may lead to hyperglycemia, and in some people with Type 1 diabetes, ketoacidosis.

If you cannot reduce or get rid of your stress, you need to learn how to work with it. The first step is to recognize some of the signs of stress—frowning, clenching teeth, twitching, tight mouth or jaw, nervous swallowing, rapid and shallow breathing, holding your breath, hunched shoulders, stiff or tight neck, tightened fists, constant tiredness, problems sleeping, rapid bounding heartbeat, and sweating.

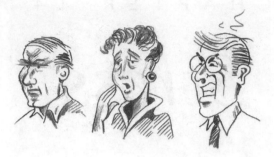

If your stress is caused by an illness, seek your doctor's help and use your sick day plan (pages 165–168).

Avoid the stress of hypoglycemia (low blood sugar) by eating meals and snacks on time; snacking when necessary before, during, or after exercise; and taking only your prescribed amount of insulin or oral medication.

EXERCISE is one of the best methods to REDUCE STRESS. It relaxes your body, changes your thoughts away from stress, lowers the blood sugar by decreasing the stress hormones, fights depression, and provides a release for the pent-up emotions. Most insurances offer help with stress through Behavioral Health (call the member services number). Check local libraries, churches, and the internet for more resources on stress management. See Chapter 10 about exercise.

Finally, if you are unable to reduce your stress, you can make a difference in the way it affects your body by using relaxation techniques. Examples of these techniques are biofeedback, guided imagery, meditation, self-hypnosis, and progressive relaxation. They require training, so ask your doctor or diabetes educator for assistance. For more information on these relaxation techniques, see *The Diabetic's Total Health and Happiness Book*, by June Biermann and Barbara Toohey (see page 205).

REMEMBER: Stress can make a difference not only in your blood sugar but also in the way you feel about yourself. Take care of YOU!

Additional sources of information on stress are

Stress without Distress, by Hans Seyle. New American Library, New York, 1975.

The Stress of Life, by Hans Seyle. McGraw, New York, 1970.

When I Say No, I Feel Guilty, by Manuel J. Smith, Ph.D. Bantam Books, New York, 1985.

Caring for the Diabetic Soul, American Diabetes Association, Alexandria, VA, 1997.

Diabetes Burnout: What to Do When You Can't Take It Anymore, by William H. Polonsky, Ph.D., C.D.E., 1999.

101 Tips for Coping with Diabetes, by Richard Rubin, Ph.D., C.D.E.; Gary M. Arsham, M.D., Ph.D.; Catherine Feste, B.A.; David G Marrero, Ph.D.; and Stefan H. Rubin.

Stress-Free Diabetes: Your Guide to Health and Happiness, by Joseph Napora, Ph.D., LCSW-C. American Diabetes Association, 2010

CHAPTER 15

Emotions— They Are a Part of Us

Any time you suffer a loss (such as losing a loved one, a job, or a friend) or are told you have a disease, all sorts of feelings or emotions are aroused—denial, anger, fear, guilt, depression. These emotions are quite normal, and everyone feels them from time to time. It is important for you to understand them, know when you are having them, and allow yourself to feel them.

The following are examples:

DENIAL—I can't believe this is happening to me. If I don't think about this, it will go away in time.

ANGER—Why me? This is not fair!

FEAR—What's going to happen to me now? I won't be able to go anywhere.

GUILT—If I hadn't eaten so much sugar, this would have never happened to me. What did I do to deserve this punishment?

DEPRESSION—I feel so alone. No one understands.

Once you work through these emotions you will reach a better understanding of your loss or disease. This is known as acceptance. You may not like, want, or be joyous about having diabetes, but at this point you will have chosen to make the necessary changes for your own good health and well-being.

ACCEPTANCE—I have diabetes now so I'm going to change my eating habits, control my blood sugar, and lose this extra weight. I'm not fond of sticking my finger, but if testing my blood sugar helps me control my diabetes, I will do it.

There is no set pattern or time limit as to how and when these emotions are felt. As sensitive, feeling people, we move back and forth through them all the time.

Emotions can actually be helpful as you grow and work toward good control of your diabetes, but each one can become a problem and disrupt not only your blood sugar control but your life, as well. How do you know when any one of these emotions might be causing you a problem? Here are some clues:

■ How long does the emotion last?

There is no time limit for an emotion, but any extreme of time is unhealthy. For a short time after being told you have diabetes, it is normal to deny or not want to think about the problem. However, if that denial is spread over years, you will be unable to control your blood sugar, and that can be dangerous for your health.

■ How strongly do you feel the emotion?

Emotions are felt in varying degrees. One day you may feel depressed and actually cry about having to give yourself an insulin injection; the next day you give the injection without a thought. It's when the depression is so strong that you don't have the energy to care for yourself or can't give the insulin injections that it becomes unhealthy.

■ Are your emotions affecting your life—relationships with family members, friends, co-workers, job, or activities?

There may be times when your feelings about diabetes do affect these aspects of your life, especially when your blood sugars are out of control or when you are first diagnosed. But use caution—don't let the diabetes be a scapegoat. Not all the problems in your life will be related to having diabetes, and some may have existed before the diabetes.

REMEMBER: It is normal to feel these emotions— just do not let them get in the way of taking care of YOU!

As you feel these emotions of denial, anger, fear, guilt, and depression from time to time, remember that they are normal and healthy. If you or someone special to you is struggling to overcome any or all of them, there are certain things you can do to work through them:

■ Have a good understanding of how each emotion makes you feel.
■ Be alert for when you, as well as your family members or significant other, are feeling these emotions.

- Use activities such as exercise, sports, and hobbies to work through these emotions.

- Choose one or two people (outside of your family) who are willing to listen when you need to talk or complain. Members of your health care team are usually quite willing to help.

- Seek out emotional support from your family, friends, clergy, and health care team. Support groups made up of others experiencing these emotions and changes can be extremely helpful.

- If the emotions are serious enough to interfere with your health and well-being, seek professional help from a counselor, social worker, or psychologist.

The following are excellent resources for more information on emotions:

Caring for the Diabetic Soul. American Diabetes Association, 1997.

Diabetes—Caring for Your Emotions as Well as Your Health, by Jerry Edelwich and Archie Brodsky. Addison-Wesley Publishing Co., Inc., Menlo Park, CA, 1998.

The Physician Within, by Catherine Feste. Henry Holt & Company, Inc., New York, 1995.

Psyching Out Your Diabetes, by June Biermann, Barbara Toohey, and Richard Rubin, PhD. Lowell House, Los Angeles, 1999.

101 Tips for Coping with Diabetes, by Richard Rubin, PhD, CDE, Gary M. Anderson, MD, PhD; Catherine Feste, BA; David G. Marrero, PhD; and Stefan H. Rubin.

1,000 Years of Diabetic Wisdom, by David G. Marrero, PhD; Robert M. Anderson, EdD; Martha M. Funnell, MS, RN, CDE; and Melinda D. Maryniuk, MED, RO, CDE. American Diabetes Association, 2008.

Behavioral Diabetes Institute—an organization that helps people overcome the emotional and behavioral obstacles of living well with diabetes. Address is P.O. Box 501866, San Diego, CA 92150-1866. Phone number is 858-336-8693. www.behavioraldiabetesinstitute.org.

CHAPTER 16

Traveling with Diabetes

Having diabetes should not limit your travel plans. Careful planning and a few special precautions can ensure a trouble-free and enjoyable trip. The following are some helpful hints to aid you in your planning.

- Have a general checkup before you leave.
- If immunizations are required, arrange to get them early in case of reactions or side effects.
- Carry some form of diabetic identification—a chain or bracelet—on your person.
- Have your doctor order a medication for you to prevent nausea and diarrhea.
- Take along 2–3 times the medication and equipment you will need—insulin, oral medications, syringes, blood and/or urine testing materials, and so on. CARRY these items WITH YOU, not in luggage that can be lost or stored in extreme temperatures.

183

- Carry a written note from your doctor stating that you have diabetes, especially if you take insulin and need to carry insulin syringes.

- Carry all of your medicines in the containers from the pharmacy. This will show the name of the medicine and that it belongs to you. If you need to take syringes, carry the prescription label from your box of syringes.

- Guidelines for traveling with insulin can change at any time. Check with your airline or the Transportation Security Administration (TSA). Call 1-866-289-9673 or www.tsa.gov/public.

- If traveling in a foreign country, learn or have written-out helpful phrases such as "I am a diabetic" and "I need a doctor."

- For information regarding diabetic care or diabetes associations in foreign countries, contact

    The International Diabetes Federation
    Avenue Emile Demot 19
    1000 Brussels, Belgium
    www.idf.org/home/

- If you will be crossing time zones, plan your insulin and medication schedule adjustments with your doctor or diabetes educator. Also think about the type of vacation you are planning—backpacking vs. driving, cross-country skiing vs. sunbathing. Check the Time Zone Converter for information on time zones across the world. www.timezoneconverter.com

- When driving for long periods, stop frequently to stretch your legs and walk.

- Carry a FAST SUGAR FOOD at all times. Also carry a snack that includes a serving from the bread and meat groups such as cheese and crackers or a peanut butter sandwich.

- The airlines can have special meals for diabetics available if you call at least two days before your flight.
- Wherever you are going, plan to arrive in the evening so you can settle in, get a good night's sleep, and start fresh in the morning.
- Check restaurant menus ahead of time so you know what they have to offer. Also avoid the dinner rush hours.
- Pay special attention to foot care, especially if you are sightseeing, hiking, or skiing.
- If you are caught in an overseas emergency, call the American embassy.

> REMEMBER: Caring for your diabetes may require extra time and planning, but do not let that stop you from going anywhere or doing anything you want!

SOURCES OF ADDITIONAL HELPFUL INFORMATION

The Peripatetic Diabetic, by June Biermann and Barbara Toohey. J.P. Tarcher, Inc., Los Angeles, 1984.

The Diabetic's Book: All Your Questions Answered, by June Biermann and Barbara Toohey. Sherbourn Press, Inc., Los Angeles, 1998.

The Joslin Guide to Diabetes, by Richard S. Beaser, M.D., with Joan V. C. Hill, R.D., C.D.E. The Joslin Center, Boston, 1995.

Directory of English-speaking Physicians throughout the World. International Association for Medical Assistance to Travelers, 417 Center Street, Lewiston, NY 14092, www.iamat.org/, (716)754-4883. A small donation is requested.

International SOS Assistance, Inc. 8 Neshaminy Interplex, #207, Trevose, PA 19053-6956, www.InternationalSOS.com, (800)523-8662.

Services include English-speaking physicians in foreign countries, and international medical and emergency care. Membership is required, and there is a fee.

The Diabetes Traveler, P.O. Box 8223 RW, Stamford, CT 06905, (203)327-5832. www.sath.org

This is a newsletter printed four times a year to help people with diabetes plan safe travel. There is an annual fee. Each issue discusses specific places such as Spain, Hawaii, Vancouver, or Paris; types of trips such as train, plane, condo vacations, or spa vacations; and other travel tips such as generic and foreign country names for drugs, travel cases, and carrying medical ID.

Centers for Disease Control and Prevention: (800)311-3435. www.cdc.gov/netinfo.htm

Travel Assistance International: (800)821-2828. www.travelassistance .com/

Traveler's Emergency Network: (800)275-4836. www.tenweb.com/

Health Information for International Travel, by the Centers for Disease Control and Prevention. Published every 2 years by the CDC as a reference for health care providers but may be useful for others. Order from the Public Health Foundation, (877)252-1200 or http://bookstore.phf .org/cat24.htm

The Diabetes Travel Guide, by Davida Kruger, M.S.N., R.N., C.S., C.D.E.

CHAPTER 17

Complications of Diabetes

High blood sugar over long periods of time damage certain tissues of the body, causing the complications of diabetes involving the eyes, kidneys, nerves, heart, and blood vessels. Research has proven that strict control of the blood sugar (in the target range the majority of the time and the Hemoglobin A1c under 7%—see page 28) can delay the onset and lessen the severity of this tissue damage.

All of your diabetes team members—doctor, diabetes nurse, dietitian, exercise specialist, and pharmacist—recommend strict control of blood sugar as your weapon against developing complications. There can be no guarantees, however; anyone with diabetes may develop one or more complications, and you should be familiar with them.

HEART AND BLOOD VESSEL DISEASE

When you have diabetes you are at greater risk for heart and blood vessel disease—which can lead to heart attack, stroke, and loss of blood supply to the legs and feet—especially if the blood sugars are out of control. Atherosclerosis (clogging of the arteries) occurs at a younger age and progresses more rapidly when blood sugars and cholesterol run high. There are 4 types of cholesterol that are measured in your blood: total cholesterol, triglycerides, HDL (good) cholesterol, and LDL (bad) cholesterol. Family history (genetics) has a lot to do with this complication. Talk to your family members to see what kind of problems they have had. Strict control of cholesterol (see page 187, Know Your Numbers) and blood sugar is a must in delaying the onset and in lessening the severity of these problems.

NERVES

Neuropathy means a change in the nerves of the body. People who have had diabetes for a long time and have poor blood sugar control may feel changes such as burning, tingling, numbness, or loss of feeling in the feet, legs, or hands; dizziness, especially when moving from a lying to a sitting or

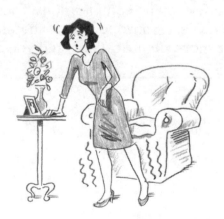

standing position; ringing or buzzing in the ears; unable to digest food correctly; gas, diarrhea, or constipation; impotence in men; decreased sexual arousal or dry vaginal walls in women; and unable to completely empty the bladder.

Strict blood sugar control—keeping blood sugars in the target range most of the time and hemoglobin A1c under 7%—has been proven to prevent or delay the onset of these problems.

EYES

Blurred vision is very common when your blood sugar is out of control—either high (hyperglycemia) or low (hypoglycemia). It will correct itself when you have regained good control of your blood sugar.

Cataracts and glaucoma may occur more often in people with diabetes.

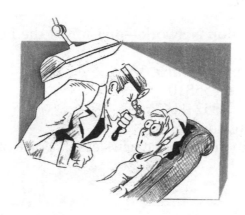

Retinopathy is the breaking and bleeding of very small blood vessels in the retina, which is located in the back of the eye. If this happens too much and is not treated, it can cause vision loss and blindness. In the early stages, you do not feel or see this happening, so REGULAR EYE EXAMS (including "dilation") ARE A MUST EACH YEAR! Strict blood sugar control—keeping blood sugars in the target range most of the time and hemoglobin A1c under 7%—has been proven to prevent or delay this complication. The earlier this problem is diagnosed, the more successful the treatment.

If you have any vision loss, you may find the following resources helpful:

The Braille Institute
741 N. Vermont Ave.
Los Angeles, CA 90029
Phone: (323) 663-1111
www.brailleinstitute.com

National Federation of the Blind
1800 Johnson St.
Baltimore, MD 21230
Phone: (410) 659-9314
www.nfb.org

Diabetes Action Network—division of the Federation of the Blind
3305 Stonebrook Circle NW
Huntsville, AL 35810
Phone: (256) 852-4143
www.nfb.org/voice.htm
Membership includes the newsletter, "Voice of the Diabetic."

KIDNEYS

Kidney and bladder infections are more of a problem when blood sugars are out of control.

After many years of having diabetes, especially if blood sugars have been out of control, the kidneys may show tissue changes that can lead to kidney damage. High blood pressure can also lead to kidney damage. Again, strict control of blood pressure and blood sugar—blood sugars in the target range most of the time and Hemoglobin A1c under 7% and blood pressure under 140/90 mm Hg—have been proven to prevent or delay the onset of this problem.

Regular checkups with your doctor are important. A urine test for microalbumin can be done to see if any tissue damage is occurring in the kidneys. If there is, you will be given a medicine to help protect your kidneys. It is important to the find these changes early on.

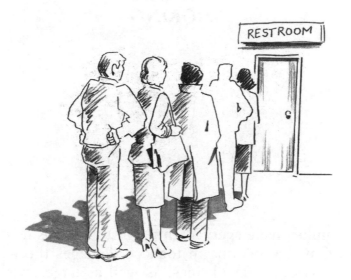

TEETH AND GUMS

If your gums are not healthy you will not only have problems with your teeth, but you may also have a hard time controlling your blood sugar. Having diabetes gives you a greater chance of having periodontal disease, especially when blood sugars have been out of control for long periods of time. Periodontal disease is redness and swelling of the gums and can include bleeding, sensitive gums, infection, and loss of teeth. It also raises your risk of heart disease, heart attacks, and stroke.

Take special care of your teeth and gums by brushing and flossing every day. See your dentist or dental hygienist for regular cleaning and checkups.

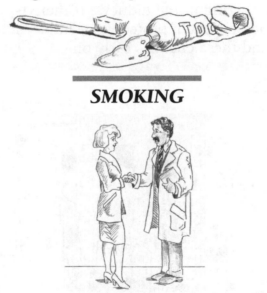

SMOKING

If you smoke, make every attempt to stop. It has now been proven that the nicotine in tobacco damages the walls of *all* blood vessels—small ones, as well as large ones. This damage results in narrowed or blocked arteries, reducing blood flow all over the body. By reducing blood flow to the body's tissues, you will increase your chances of getting one or more of the complications of diabetes or of worsening any of those you may already have.

REMEMBER: Good control of your blood sugars will prevent, delay, or lessen the severity of the complications of diabetes.

See your doctor regularly and make sure you have the following tests and checkups:

- Estimated Average Glucose (eAG) (Hemoglobin A1c) every 3–6 months
- Cholesterol, Triglycerides, HDL and LDL every year (check with your doctor if they are not normal)
- Blood pressure checked each visit
- Urine for microalbumin yearly
- Eyes checked (with dilation) yearly
- Dental check/cleaning twice a year
- Feet checked at least yearly

KNOW YOUR NUMBERS: Ask your doctor for the results of your tests and compare them with the target ranges to see how well you are doing.

- Estimated Average
  Glucose (eAG)—Goal: under 140–154)*
  Hemoglobin A1c—Goal: under 6.5%–7%*
  *But these goals may need to be adjusted for you with your health care provider.
- Blood Pressure—Goal: under 140/90 mmHg
- Cholesterol—Goal:
  Total cholesterol—under 200 mg/dl
  Triglycerides—under 150 mg/dl
  HDL—over 40 mg/dl in men over 50 mg/dl in women
  LDL—under 100mg/dl (for some people,under 70)

The most important thing you can do is take proper care of yourself—that means eating the right foods, taking the right amount of medicine, testing your blood sugar, and exercising.

Research on Diabetes

Diabetes mellitus is a disease that has been known to man for approximately 3,000–4,000 years. After all this time, the cause of diabetes still remains a mystery, and modern medicine has not yet been able to provide a cure. Researchers all over the world are busily seeking out the cause of and a cure for diabetes, as well as developing devices to help diabetics maintain better control of their blood sugars.

For Type 1 diabetes, research is centered on

- Pancreas transplants (whole, partial, and islet cell)
- Developing an implantable artificial pancreas (similar to a pacemaker) that can measure blood sugar and provide insulin according to the body's needs
- Improving the presently available insulin pumps (see page 147) to make them smaller, lighter, and easier to operate
- Studying the human body's immune system (the body's ability to fight against foreign tissue, bacteria, viruses, and so on)
- Developing a way to prevent the onset of Type 1 diabetes

- Developing an insulin pump and glucose sensor (to measure the blood sugar) that can be placed inside the body
- Developing medicines to prevent the body from destroying the cells of the pancreas that make insulin
- Developing a way to give insulin other than by injection

For Type 2 diabetes, research is centered on

- The causes of obesity
- Safe and effective ways to reduce weight—programs that include behavior modification and support groups such as Weight Watchers and Over-Eaters Anonymous
- Safe and effective ways to control appetite
- Developing more effective oral medications
- Why certain groups of people (Native Americans, Asian Americans, African Americans, and Hispanic Americans) are more likely to have Type 2 diabetes
- Ways to make the fat and muscle cells more sensitive to insulin

For both Type 1 and Type 2 diabetes, research is focused on

- Studying the function and malfunction of glucagon (another hormone produced by the pancreas) that works the opposite of insulin
- The effects and benefits of exercise
- The makeup, combination, breakdown, and absorption of various foods and their effects on blood sugar
- Stress—its effects on the body and ways to reduce it using behavior modification and relaxation techniques
- Finding ways to make pregnancy safe for both the mother and the baby

- Understanding the cause of the complications of diabetes and better ways to treat them
- Developing other ways to give insulin—orally, nasally, and in eye drops
- Developing easier ways to check blood sugar

Research is changing diabetes care and management for both Type 1 and Type 2 diabetes very rapidly. The best way to keep in touch with the new changes is to read *Diabetes Forecast, Diabetes Self-Management,* and *Diabetes Health.* See page 200 for information on these magazines.

CHAPTER 19

Organizations and Resources

Your local chapter of the American Diabetes Association is actively involved in many different programs. It is concerned with public education, helps provide research grants, and sponsors outpatient education programs.

If you would like additional information about diabetes, you are welcome to contact any of the offices of the American Diabetes Association. Call or write for the office closest to you:

American Diabetes Association
1701 N. Beauregard St.
Alexandria, VA 22311
(800)342-2383
www.diabetes.org

http://shopdiabetes.org is the website for the bookstore of the American Diabetes Association.

Juvenile Diabetes Research Foundation International
26 Broadway
New York, NY 10004
(800)JDF-CURE (533-2873)
www.jdrf.org

Taking Control of Your Diabetes
1110 Camino Del Mar, Suite B
Del Mar, CA 92014
(800) 99TCOYD (800-998-2693)
www.tcoyd.org

Journey for Control
Λ program from Merck to help you understand, live with,
and manage diabetes.
www.journeyforcontrol.com

You will also be able to keep abreast of all the new ideas
and products, as well as review your present knowledge of
diabetes, by reading any of the following magazines:

Diabetes Forecast Magazine
American Diabetes Association, Inc.
1701 N. Beauregard St.
Alexandria, VA 22311
(800) 806-7801
This is also printed in Spanish.

Diabetes Self-Management
Phone: (855) 367-4813
Fax: (617) 536-0102
www.diabetesselfmanagement.com

Diabetes Health
365 Bel Marin Keys Blvd., #100
Novato, CA 94949
(415) 883-1990
www.diabeteshealth.com

To find a certified diabetes educator (CDE) nurse, dietician, or pharmacist near you:

- Check the hospitals, medical groups, and pharmacies in your area.

- Check with the American Association of Diabetes Educators at www.diabeteseducator.org or (800) 338-3633.

- Check with the American Diabetes Association at www.diabetes.org or (800) 342-2383.

WEB PAGE ADDRESSES

About Health and Fitness:
www.diabetes-about.com

American Association of Diabetes Educators:
www.diabeteseducator.org

American Diabetes Association: www.diabetes.org

The American Diabetes Association Bookstore:
www.shopdiabetes.org

The American Dietetic Association:
www.eatright.org

Behavioral Diabetes Institute:
www. behavioraldiabetesinstitute.org

Canadian Diabetes Association: www.diabetes.ca

Children with Diabetes:
www.childrenwithdiabetes.com

Diabetes and More:
Source for diabetes products:
www.diabetesandmore.com

Diabetes Mall on Diabetes Net:
www.diabetesnet.com

The Diabetes Monitor:
www.diabetesmonitor.com

Diabetes Self-Management:
www.diabetesselfmanagement.com

Food and Nutrition Information Center:
www.nalusda.gov/fnic

International Diabetes Federation: www.idf.org

Joslin Diabetes Center: www.joslin.org

Juvenile Diabetes Research Foundation International:
www.jdrf.org

Medline Plus:
www.medlineplus.gov

The Merck Journey for Control Program:
www.journeyforcontrol.com

My Health Advisor
www.diabetes.org/mha

National Diabetes Education Program:
www.ndep.nih.gov

National Institutes of Health (NIH):
www.nlm.nih.gov/medlineplus

WebMD
Quality health information and services: www.webmd.com

APPS FOR DIABETES

Here are several helpful apps. There are many more
available and new ones being developed.

Diabetes Meal from Everyday Health

GluCoMo   Records blood sugars, insulin, and other
           health information

Go Meals   Uses the plate method to plan meals. Includes
           nutrition facts of foods and restaurant meals.

Calorie King	Provides the calories, carbohydrate, and fat content of foods and restaurant menu items.
Fooducate	Scan barcodes or search for food nutrition facts.
Weight Watchers Mobile	Weight Watchers diet plan; information about local meetings.
Diabetes Pilot	Records blood sugars, insulin and other medicines, food, exercise, blood pressure, and weight. Can provide information on nutrition facts and restaurants.
Diabetes Pal	Logs blood sugars, medicine, and food. Allows you to add notes.
Blue Loop	Records, stores, and shares diabetes information in real time.
Log Frog Diabetes	Logs your blood sugars; simple and fun.
Glucose Buddy	Records your blood sugars, medicines, food, and exercise. Can set reminders to test your blood sugar.
Med Simple	Tracks medicines—prescription and over-the-counter. Can set alerts to remind you to take your medicines.
Blood Sugar Tracker	Allows you to set your own blood sugar target ranges and view simple graphs of history of blood sugars to see patterns.
Zombies Run	Fitness game that combines exercize training with a zombie story.
GAIN	Allows you to coordinate your exercise routines (time and available equipment) with your fitness goals.

iTreadmill	Tracks your steps, distance, and speed.
iFitness	Helps you find the right exercise for the right muscles. Videos available with tips on technique.
GymGoalABC	Teaches weight lifting
Fitness Builder	Has over 800 workouts and 6,000 images and videos to see. You can build your own workouts.
Run Keeper	Records your distance, time, and calories burned while doing a variety of activities.

dLife TV

dLife TV has moved online at www.dLifeTV.com. Tune in Sundays at 7:00 p.m. (ET)/4:00 p.m. (PT)

You can also visit the website at www.dlife.com where you will find the latest diabetes medical news, stories from people living with diabetes, and many recipes. Become a member (free) and access recipes, food information, newsletters, community forums, and expert answers to questions.

BOOKS

Many books written about diabeties seem timeless, yet others are quickly out of date. The following books have remained interesting and helpful despite their publication dates.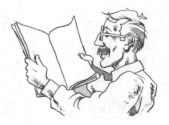

Diabetes—Caring for Your Emotions as Well as Your Health, by Jerry Edelwich and Archie Brodsky. Addison-Wesley, Menlo Park, CA, 1986.

The Diabetes Sports and Exercise Book, by Claudia Graham, C.D.E., Ph.D., M.P.H., June Biermann, and Barbara Toohey. Lowell House, Los Angeles, 1995.

The Diabetic Man, by Peter Lodewick, M.D., June Biermann, and Barbara Toohey. Lowell House, Los Angeles, 1999.

The Diabetic Woman, by Lois Jovanovic-Peterson, M.D., June Biermann, and Barbara Toohey. J.P. Tarcher, Inc., Los Angeles, 2000.

The Diabetic's Book: All Your Questions Answered, by June Biermann and Barbara Toohey. Sherbourn Press, Inc., Los Angeles, 1998.

The Diabetic's Total Health and Happiness Book, by June Biermann and Barbara Toohey. J.P. Tarcher/Penguin, Los Angeles, 2003.

The Peripatetic Diabetic, by June Biermann and Barbara Toohey. J.P. Tarcher, Inc., Los Angeles, 1984.

The Physician Within—Taking Care of Your Well-Being, by Catherine Feste. Henry Holt and Company, Inc., New York, 1995.

Psyching Out Diabetes, by June Biermann, Barbara Toohey, and Richard R. Rubin, Ph.D. Lowell House, Los Angeles, 1999.

Type II Diabetes and What to Do, by Virginia Valentine, R.N., M.S., C.D.E., June Bierman, and Barbara Toohey. Lowell House, Los Angeles, 2000.

Guide to Herbs and Nutritional Supplements: What You Need to Know from Aloe to Zinc, by Laura Shane-McWhorter C.D.E., PharmD, B.C.P.S., F.A.S.C.P, B.C.-A.D.M, C.D.E. American Diabetes Association, 2009

Everyone Likes to Eat, by Hugo J. Hollerorth, Ed.D., and Debra Kaplan, R.D., M.S. Chronimed Publishing, Minneapolis, 1993.

Transitions in Care: Meeting the Challenges of Type 1 Diabetes in Young Adults, by Howard A. Wolpert M.D., Barbara J. Anderson Ph.D., and Jill Weissberg-Benchell, Ph.D., C.D.E. American Diabetes Association, 2009

Check these resources for the most current books on diabetes And don't forget your local library.

American Diabetes Association
1701 N. Beauregard St.
Alexandria, VA 22311
www.diabetes.org or (800) 342-2383.

The Joslin Center for Diabetes
One Joslin PLace
Boston, MA 02215
www.joslin.org or (617) 309-2400

Juvenile Diabetes Research Foundation International
26 Broadway
New York, NY 10004
www.jdrf.org or (800)JDF-CURE (533-2873)

The Diabetes Mall
1030 Upas Street
San Diego, CA 92103
www.diabetesnet.com or (800) 998-4772

International Diabetes Center
3800 Park Nicollet Blvd.
Minneapolis, MN 55416-2699
www.idcpublishing.com or (800) 637-2675

www.amazon.com

Answers to Quiz on Hyperglycemia and Hypoglycemia

(page 24)

1.
a. hyper
b. hypo
c. both
d. hyper
e. hyper
f. hyper
g. hyper
h. hypo

i. hyper
j. hyper
k. hypo
l. hypo
m. both (more often hyper)
n. hypo

2.
a
ⓑ
ⓒ
d
ⓔ
ⓕ

Meal-Planning Forms

On the following pages you will find blank Meal Planning Forms. Make as many copies of them as you desire. Use them to plan your meals. Bring them along when you see your dietitian or diabetes educator.

Personalized Meal Plan

Number of Calories: _____

Carbohydrate: _____ grams Protein: _____ grams

Fat: _____ grams

Breakfast Time: _____

_____ Carbohydrate Choices

    _____ starch

    _____ fruit

    _____ milk

_____ Meat Choices

_____ Fat Choices

Morning Snack Time: _____

_____

Lunch Time: _____

_____ Carbohydrate Choices

    _____ starch

    _____ fruit

    _____ milk

_____ Vegetables

_____ Meat Choices

_____ Fat Choices

Afternoon Snack Time: _____

_____

Dinner Time: _____

_____ Carbohydrate Choices

    _____ starch

    _____ fruit

    _____ milk

_____ Vegetables

_____ Meat Choices

_____ Fat Choices

Evening Snack Time: _____

_____

Personalized Meal Plan

Number of Calories: _____

Carbohydrate: _____ grams Protein: _____ grams

Fat: _____ grams

Breakfast Time: _____

_____ Carbohydrate Choices

_____ starch

_____ fruit

_____ milk

_____ Meat Choices

_____ Fat Choices

Morning Snack Time: _____

_____

Lunch Time: _____

_____ Carbohydrate Choices

_____ starch

_____ fruit

_____ milk

_____ Vegetables

_____ Meat Choices

_____ Fat Choices

Afternoon Snack Time: _____

_____

Dinner Time: _____

_____ Carbohydrate Choices

_____ starch

_____ fruit

_____ milk

_____ Vegetables

_____ Meat Choices

_____ Fat Choices

Evening Snack Time: _____

_____

Personalized Meal Plan

Number of Calories: _____

Carbohydrate: _____ grams   Protein: _____ grams

Fat: _____ grams

Breakfast Time: _____

_____ Carbohydrate Choices
  _____ starch
  _____ fruit
  _____ milk
_____ Meat Choices
_____ Fat Choices

Morning Snack Time: _____

_____

Lunch Time: _____

_____ Carbohydrate Choices
  _____ starch
  _____ fruit
  _____ milk
_____ Vegetables
_____ Meat Choices
_____ Fat Choices

Afternoon Snack Time: _____

_____

Dinner Time: _____

_____ Carbohydrate Choices
  _____ starch
  _____ fruit
  _____ milk
_____ Vegetables
_____ Meat Choices
_____ Fat Choices

Evening Snack Time: _____

_____

APPENDIX C

Bibliography

American Diabetes Association, *The Diabetes Food & Nutrition Bible.* American Diabetes Association, Alexandria, VA, 2003.

American Diabetes Association, *Footcare for the Diabetic,* Association handout.

American Diabetes Association, *Complete Guide To Diabetes*, American Diabetes Association, Alexandria, VA, 2005

American Diabetes Association, "Nutrition Recommendations and Principles for People with Diabetes Mellitus." *Diabetes Care* 21, suppl. 1, 1998.

American Diabetes Association/American Dietetic Association, *Exchange Lists for Meal Planning.* American Diabetes Association/ American Dietetic Association, 2003.

Biermann, June, and Barbara Toohey, *The Peripatetic Diabetic.* J.P. Tarcher, Los Angeles, 1984.

Biermann, June, Barbara Toohey, and Claudia Graham, DCE, Ph.D., MPH, *The Diabetic's Sports and Exercise Book*. Lowell House, Los Angeles, 1995.

Binney, Ruth, ed., *The Complete Manual of Fitness and Well-Being.* Viking Penguin, New York, 1984.

Chaney, Patricia S., ed., *Managing Diabetics Properly.* Nursing 77 Skillbook Series, Intermed Communications, Horsham, PA, 1977.

"Clinical Practice Recommendations." *Diabetes Care*, volume 29, supplement 1, 2006.

"Clinical Practice Recommendations." *Diabetes Care*, volume 36, supplement 1, January, 2013.

Cooper, Kenneth, M.D., M.P.H., *Aerobics Program for Total Well-Being: Exercise, Diet, Emotional Balance*. M. Evans, New York, 1982.

Cooper, Kenneth, M.D., M.P.H., *The Aerobics Way*. Bantam Books, New York, 1977.

Davidson, Mayer B., *Diabetes Mellitus: Diagnosis and Treatment*, 4th edition. W.B. Saunders, Philadelphia, 1998.

"Diabetes Apps," *Diabetes Forecast*, January 2013.

Edelwich, Jerry, and Archie Brodsky, *Diabetes: Caring for Your Emotions as Well as Your Health*. Addison-Wesley, Menlo Park, CA, 1986.

Franz, M. J., et al., "Nutrition Principles for the Management of Diabetes and Related Complications." *Diabetes Care*, May 1994.

Gilmore, C. P., *Exercise for Fitness*. Time Life Books, Alexandria, VA, 1981.

Guthrie, Diane, RN, Ph.D., and Richard A. Guthrie, M.D., *The Diabetes Sourcebook*. Lowell House, Los Angeles, 1997.

Guyton, Arthur, C., M.D., *Function of the Human Body*. W.B. Saunders, Philadelphia, 1985.

Hodge, Robert H., Jr., M.D., et al., "Multiple Use of Disposable Insulin Syringe-Needle Units." *JAMA*, 244, no. 3, 1980.

Holler, H. J., and J. G. Pastors, eds., *Meal Planning Approaches for Diabetes Management*. American Dietetic Association, Chicago, 1994.

Holzmeister, Lea Ann. R.D., C.D.E., *The Diabetic Carbohydrate and Fat Gram Guide*, The American Diabetes Association, Alexandria, VA. 2005

Jornsay, Donna L., R.N., BSN, CPNP, CDE, and Daniel L. Lorber, M.D., "Diabetes and the Traveler." *Clinical Diabetes*, 6, no. 3, May/June 1988, pp. 52–55.

Kübler-Ross, Elizabeth, M.D., *On Death and Dying*. Macmillan, New York, 1969.

Lasker, Roz D., M.D. "The Effect of Intensive Treatment of Diabetes on the Development and Progression of Long-Term Complications in Insulin-Dependent Diabetes Mellitus." *New England Journal of Medicine*, 14, no. 329, Sept. 30, 1993, pp. 977–1036.

Leontos, Carolyn, M.S., R.D., C.D.E., Geil, Pattie, M.S., R.D., .A.D.A., C.D.E., *Individualized Approaches to Diabetes Nutrition Therapy.* American Diabetes Association, Alexandria, VA. 2005

Middleton, Katherine, and May Abbott Hess, *The Art of Cooking for the Diabetic*, 3rd edition. Contemporary Books, Chicago, 1997.

Peragallo-Dittko, Virginia, R.N., M.A., C.D.E., ed., *A Core Curriculum for Diabetes Education*, 3rd edition. American Association of Diabetes Educators, Chicago, 1998.

Rafkin-Mervis, Lisa E., M.S., R.D., "Carbohydrate Counting." *Diabetes Forecast*, Feb. 1995, pp. 30–37.

"Standards of Care–Position Statement." *Diabetes Care*, 26, supplement 1, January 2003, page 538.

"Standards of Medical Care in Diabetes 2015," *Diabetes Care*, 38, supplement 1, January 2015.

Sutherland, David, M.D., PhD., et al., "Pancreas Transplantation—A Historical Overview and Its Current Status." *The Diabetes Educator*, 1, Spring 1982, pp. 11–13.

"Syringe Reuse." *Diabetes Care*, 8, no. 1, Jan.–Feb. 1985, pp. 97–99.

Torregiani, Seth, "Untangling the Net." *Diabetes Self-Management*, July–August 1997, pp. 22–28.

"The United Kingdom Prospective Diabetes Study (UKPDS) for Type 2 Diabetes." *Lancet*, 352, 1998, pp. 837–852.

Vessby, B., "Dietary Carbohydrates and Diabetes." *American Journal of Clinical Nutrition*, March 1994.

Warshaw, Hope, R.D., C.D.E., *Diabetes Meal Planning Made Easy*, 2nd edition. American Diabetes Association, Alexandria, VA. 2005

"Translating the A1c Assay Into Estimated Average Glucose Values," *Diabetes Care*, 31, no. 8, August 2008, pp. 1–6.

Index

Note: Page numbers followed by "f" indicate figures; those followed by "t" indicate tables.

Academy of Nutrition and Dietetics, referral service, 107
Acarbose (Precose), 128t
Acceptance, 180
Acesulfame-K, 82
Acetest, 121
Acetohexamide (Dymelor), 124t
Acetone. *See* Ketones
Activity. *See also* Exercise
  age and, 33
  causing blood sugar fluctuation, 37t
  weight and, 32, 33
Actos (Pioglitazone), 127t
Actos plus Met, 131t
Aerobic exercise, 154, 156
Age, activity and, 33
Albiglutide (Tanzeum), 133t, 134
Alcohol, 154
  cooking with, 89
  diet plan, 89
  use of, 88–89
Alfrezza, 136t
Alogliptin (Nesina), 129t
Alpha-glucosidase inhibitors, 128–129, 128t
Alternative meals, 76
Alternative sweeteners, 82, 83
Amaryl (Glimepiride), 124t

American Association of Diabetes Education, 201
American Diabetes and Dietetic Associations, 37
American Diabetes Association, 103, 173, 199, 201
Amylin mimetic, 134, 134t
Anaerobic exercise, 154
Anger, 179
Apidra, 136t, 142
Appetite control, 196
Apps, 202–204
Aspartame, 82
At risk for diabetes, 6
Avandamet, 131t
Avandaryl, 131t
Avandia (Rosiglitazone), 127t

Beans, 46
Biguanides, 126–127, 126t
Blood fat target, 100
Blood glucose. *See* Blood sugar
Blood pressure, high, 32
Blood sugar, 7–9, 14, 39–40. *See also* Blood sugar levels; Blood sugar tests
  balanced, 26
  low, 18

Blood sugar levels
  activities causing fluctuation, 27t
  causes of fluctuations, 26–28t
  diet causing fluctuation, 27t
  emotions causing fluctuation, 27t
  insulin causing fluctuation,
    26–27t
  oral medication causing
    fluctuation, 26–27t
  patterns of, 115
  sickness causing fluctuation, 28t
  target/acceptable ranges, 28
  target range, 28t
  testing, 28
Blood sugar tests
  chart, 118t
  estimated average glucose,
    150–152
  fasting blood sugar, 149
  helpful hints, 114–117
  at home, 111–114
  improving through research, 197
  laboratory tests, 149–152
  post-prandial, 149–150
  record keeping, 115
Blood vessel disease complica?tions,
  188
BMI, 34–36, 35t
  calculation of, 36
Body mass index. See BMI
Books on diabetes, 204–206
Borderline diabetes. See At risk for
  diabetes
Bread, 43–44
Bydureon (Exenatide extended
  release), 133t, 134
Byetta (Exenatide), 133t

Cake-decorating gel, 19
Calories
  1500 sample meals plans, 79t

2000 sample meals plans, 80t–81t
  consumption of, 33–34
  on food labels, 85
Canagliflozin (Invokana), 130t
Carbohydrate Group, 37
Carbohydrates, 7, 8
  blood glucose and, 39–40
  in common foods, 167t–168t
  counting, 38–39, 39t
  meal planning and, 43–57
Cardiovascular diseases, 188
Cataracts, 189
Cereal, 44
Certified diabetes educator (CDE)
  nurses, 201
Checkups, importance of, 193
Chemstrip K, 121
Chlorpropamide (Diabinese), 124t,
  125
Cholesterol, 86, 99–101
Clear insulin, 142
Cloudy insulin, 142
Coma, diabetic. See Hyperglycemia
Combination food choices, 65–66,
  66t–67t
Combination medication, 131t–132t
Complications
  blood vessel diseases, 188
  dental problems, 192
  eye problems, 189–190
  heart diseases, 188
  kidney problems, 191
  nerve problems, 188–189
  research about, 197
  smoking issues, 192
Condiments, 72–73
Cookbooks, 34
Cooking, with alcohol, 89
Cool-down exercise, 156
Crackers, 45

Daily value, percent on food labels, 86
Dapagliflozin (Farxiga), 130t
Denial, 179
Dental complications, 192
Depression, 180
Dex Glucose Gel, 20
Diabeta (Micronase/Glyburide), 124t
Diabetes control circle, x
Diabetes Forecast Magazine, 197, 200
Diabetes Health, 197, 200
Diabetes mellitus
    complications of, 188–192
    derivation of, 1
    gestational, 6
    glucose role of, 7–9
    heredity and, 2
    immune system and, 2–3
    insulin role of, 9–10
    nutrition and, 3
    obesity and, 3
    risks for, 6
    type 1, 4
    type 2, 5
Diabetes Plate, healthy, 69, 70f, 71t
Diabetes Self-Management, 197, 200
Diabetes team, 11f
Diabetic coma. See Hyperglycemia
Diabetic emergency, 121
Diabetic keto-acidosis. See Keto-acidosis
Diabinese (Chlorpropamide), 88, 124t, 125
Diet, 29–109, 88. See also Meal planning; specific types of foods and nutrients
    alcohol, 88–89
    alternative sweeteners, 82–83
    calories, 33–34
    causing blood sugar fluctuation, 27t
    cholesterol, 99–101

dining out in restaurants, 90–99
food amount, 33–34
food choices, 42–76
healthy weight, 34–36
meal planning, 37–41
for overweight, 31–32
sample meal plans, 77–81
saturated fat, 99–101
shopping tips for food, 89–90
for type 1 diabetes, 31
for type 2 diabetes, 31–32
Dietary Guidelines for Americans, 30
Diet cookbooks, 34
Dietetic food choices, 75–76
Dietitians, referral service, 107
Dining out
    fast foods, 93–95
    in restaurants, 90–99
    suggestions, 92–93
    what not to eat, 92t
    what to eat, 91t
Diseases. See specific diseases and kinds of diseases
dLife TV, 204
DPP-4 inhibitor, 129, 129t
Drinks, 50, 72–73. See also Alcohol
Dulaglutide (Trulicity), 133t, 134
Dymelor (Acetohexamide), 124t

EAG. See Estimated average glucose (eAG)
Eating, guide to healthy, 29
Emergency, diabetic, 121
Emotions, 179–182
    Acceptance, 180
    Anger, 179
    causing blood sugar fluctuation, 27t
    Denial, 179
    Depression, 180
    Fear, 179

Empagliflozin (Jardiance), 130*t*
Equal. *See* Aspartame
Equivalents, 34
Estimated Average Glucose (eAG),
    28, 150–152
Estimated Average Glucose (eAG)
    test, 150–152
Ethnicity, 196
Exchange lists. *See* Food Choices
Exenatide (Byetta), 133*t*
Exercise, 156–160
    aerobic, 154, 156
    anaerobic, 154
    benefits of, 153–154
    consistency in, 160
    cool-down, 156
    guidelines, 162–163
    heart rate measurement and,
        156–160
    indications to stop, 161
    isometric, 154
    isotonic, 154
    to reduce stress, 176
    research about, 196
    sources of information about,
        163–164
    stretching, 155
    timing of, 160–161
    training, 156
    warm-up, 155
Eye checkups, 189
Eye complications, 189–190

Farxiga (Dapagliflozin), 130*t*
Fast foods, 93–95, 95*t*–98*t*
Fasting blood sugar range, 28
Fasting blood sugar test, 149
Fasting glucose, impaired. *See* At
    risk for diabetes
Fast sugar foods, 18, 20, 184
Fat choices, 63–65
Fat-free milk, 52

Fats, 8, 9, 40–41, 41*f*, 100–101
    high-fat meat, 62–63
    medium-fat meat, 61–62
    monounsaturated, 41, 64
    polyunsaturated, 41, 64
    saturated, 41, 65
    starch foods prepared with fat,
        46–47
    trans, 30, 41, 100
FDA. *See* Food and Drug
    Administration (FDA)
Fear, 179
Fiber, 32, 102–106
    counting, 103, 103*f*
    on food labels, 86
    in fruits, 104*t*
    in grains, 105*t*
    high-fiber diet, 106*t*
    in legumes, 105*t*
    in nuts, 106*t*
    in seeds, 106*t*
    sources of, 104*t*–106*t*
    in starches, 105*t*
    in vegetables, 104*t*–105*t*
Food amount. *See* Food portions
Food and Drug Administration
    (FDA), 84
Food choices
    alternative meals, 76
    carbohydrates, 43–57
    fruit choices, 47–50
    milk choices, 51–52
    others, 52–55
    starch choices, 43–47
    vegetable choices, 55–57
    combination foods, 65–66, 66*t*–67*t*
    dietetic foods, 75–76
    fats, 63–65
    free foods, 67–68
    guide to healthy, 29
    meats, 67–68
    high-fat meat, 62–63

lean meat, 60–61
   medium-fat meat, 61–62
   very lean meat, 58–59
Food labels, 34, 84–87, 84*t*–85*t*,
   87*f*
   calories, 85
   cholesterol, 86
   daily value percentages, 86
   fiber, 86
   protein, 86
   reading, 85–86
   serving sizes, 85
   sodium, 86
   total carbohydrate, 86
   total fat, 86
Food measurement, 33–34
   equivalents, 34
Food portions, 8–9, 33–34
   eating smaller, 32
Food shopping, tips for, 89–90
Foot care, 171–172, 171*t*–172*t*
Foot powder, 172
Fortamet (Metformin), 126*t*
Free food choices, 67–68
Fruit juice, 50
Fruits, 47–50, 104*t*

Gestational diabetes, 6. *See also*
   Pregnancy
Glaucoma, 189
Glimepiride (Amaryl), 124*t*
Glipizide (Glucotrol), 124*t*, 125
Glipizide ER (Glucotrol XL), 124*t*
Glucagon, 21, 196
GlucoBurst Gel, 20
Glucophage (Metformin), 88,
   126–127, 126*t*
Glucophage XR (Metformin ER),
   126–127, 126*t*
Glucose, 7–9. *See also* Blood sugar
Glucose gels, 19–20
Glucose meters, 112, 113*f*

Glucose Rapid Spray, 20
Glucose sensor, 196
Glucose tablets, 19–20
Glucose tolerance, impaired. *See* At
   risk for diabetes
Glucotrol (Glipizide), 124*t*, 125
Glucotrol XL (Glipizide ER), 124*t*
Glucovance, 131*t*
Glumetza (Metformin), 126*t*
Glutose, 19
Glyburide (Micronase/Diabeta), 124*t*
Glynase (Micronized Glyburide), 124*t*
Glyset (Miglitol), 128*t*
Glyxambi, 131*t*
Grains, 44–45, 105*t*
Grazing, 74
Guide to healthy eating, 29
Guilt, 179
Gums. *See* Dental complications;
   Periodontal disease

HDL cholesterol, 100
Healthy Diabetes Plate, 69, 70*f*, 71*t*
Healthy eating, 30, 41
   guide to, 29
Healthy weight, 34–36
Heart disease, 188
Heart rate
   measurement of, 156–160
   target, 156–164, 158*t*
Hemoglobin A1c, 28, 152. *See also*
   Estimated Average Glucose
   (eAG)
Heredity, 2
High blood pressure, 32
High blood sugar. *See*
   Hyperglycemia
High-fat meat, 62–63
High-fiber diet, 106*t*
High versus low blood sugar, 26–28.
   See also Hyperglycemia;
   Hypoglycemia

Home blood-sugar testing, 111–117
Home remedies, avoiding, 152
Humalog, 135*t*, 142
Humalog Mix, 135*t*
Humulin N, 135*t*
Humulin R, 135*t*
Hygiene
    foot care, 171–172
    skin care, 170
Hyperglycemia, 187
    stress and, 175–176
    symptoms of, 13–14
Hypoglycemia, 15–23, 18
    nighttime, 16
    reasons for, 16
    symptoms of, 16–17

Immune system, 2–3, 195
Impaired fasting glucose. *See* At risk
    for diabetes
Impaired glucose tolerance. *See* At
    risk for diabetes
Incretin mimetic, 133–134, 133*t*
Inhaled Insulin, 136*t*
Injected medicines. *See* Glucagon;
    Insulin
Injections
    glucagon, 21
    injection areas, 146–147
    injection timings, 138
    insulin, 9–10, 134–148
    insulin pen, 144
    insulin pumps, 147–148
    single insulin, 140–142
    techniques, 145–147
Injection technique, double insulin,
    142–144
Insta Glucose, 19
Insulin, 9–10, 134–143
    Alfrezza, 136*t*
    Apidra, 136*t*, 142

    causing blood sugar fluctuation,
        26*t*–27*t*
    clear insulin, 142
    cloudy insulin, 142
    Humalog, 135*t*, 142
    Humalog Mix, 135*t*
    Humulin N, 135*t*
    Humulin R, 135*t*
    important information, 137
    improving delivery through
        research, 197
    information to remember, 137
    inhaled, 136*t*
    injection techniques, 140–144
    injection timings, 138
    insulin pens, 144
    insulin pumps, 147–148, 195,
        196
    insulin reaction, 120 (*see also*
        Hypoglycemia)
    insulin resistance, 3, 11
    insulin shock (*see* Hypoglycemia)
    Lantus, 136*t*, 142
    Levemir, 136*t*, 142
    Lilly Insulin, 135*t*
    Novolin 70/30, 136*t*
    Novolin N, 136*t*
    Novolog, 136*t*, 142
    Novolog Mix, 136*t*
    Novolog N, 136*t*
    Novolog R, 136*t*
    Novo Nordisk, 136*t*
    Regular, 142
    reusing syringes, 140–141, 141*f*
    Sanofi, 136*t*
    storage, 138
    syringes, 139–141, 139*f*, 141*f*
    Toujeo, 136*t*
    using one type, 140–142
    using two types, 142–144
Insulin-dependent diabetes. *See* Type
    1 diabetes

Insulin pens, 144
Insulin pumps, 147–148, 195, 196
Insulin reaction, 120. *See also*
    Hypoglycemia
Insulin resistance, 3, 11
Insulin shock. *See* Hypoglycemia
Insulin storage, 138
Insulin syringes, 100–101
    buying, 140*f*
    disposing of, 145
    parts, 139*f*
    reusing, 139
International Diabetes Federation,
    184
Invokamet, 132*t*
Invokana (Canagliflozin), 130*t*
Isometric exercise, 154
Isotonic exercise, 154

Janumet, 131*t*
Janumet XR, 132*t*
Januvia (Sitagliptin), 129*t*
Jardiance (Empagliflozin), 130*t*
Jentadueto, 132*t*
Juice, 50
Juvenile diabetes. *See* Type 1
    diabetes
Juvenile Diabetes Research
    Foundation International, 200

Kazano, 132*t*
Keto-acidosis, diabetic, 119–121
Ketones, 14, 119–121
    guidelines for testing, 116, 120
Ketostix, 121, 121*f*
Kidney complications, 191
Kombliglyze XR, 131*t*

Labels. *See* Food labels
Laboratory tests, 193
    blood sugar estimated average
        glucose, 150–152

fasting blood sugar, 149
post-prandial blood sugar,
    149–150
Lancet devices, 113*f*
Lantus, 136*t*, 142
LDL cholesterol, 100
Lean meat, 58–59, 60–61
Legumes, 105*t*
Lentils, 46
Levemir, 136*t*, 142
Lilly Insulin, 135*t*
Linagliptin (Tradjenta), 129*t*
Liquid Shot, 20
Liraglutide (Victoza), 133*t*
Live Life gel, 20
Log book, 116
Low blood sugar. *See* Hypoglycemia
Low-fat crackers, 45
Low-fat snacks, 45

Maturity onset diabetes. *See* Type 2
    diabetes
Meal planning, 37–41. *See also* Diet
    beans, 46
    blood sugar and, 39–40
    bread, 43–44
    carbohydrates and, 38–39, 43–57
    cereal, 44
    combination food choices, 65–66
    condiments, 72–73
    crackers, 45
    dietetic food choices, 75–76
    drinks, 72–73
    fat choices, 40–41, 63–65
    fat-free milk, 52
    food choices, 40–41
    alternative meals, 82
    carbohydrates, 43–57
    combination foods, 65–66,
        66*t*–67*t*
    dietetic foods, 75–76
    fats, 63–65

Meal planning (*continued*)
   free foods, 67–68
   free food choices, 67–68
   fruit choices, 47–50
   grains, 44–45
   healthy Diabetes Plate, 69, 70*f*,
      71*t*
   high-fat meat, 62–63
   lean meat, 60–61
   lentils, 46
   low-fat crackers, 45
   low-fat snacks, 45
   meat choices, 57–63, 58*t*
   medium-fat meat, 61–62
   milk choices, 51–52
   pasta, 44–45
   peas, 46
   plate method, 69, 70*f*, 71*t*
   proteins, 40
   resources, 107
   seasonings, 73–74
   snacks, 45
   starch choices, 43–47
   starchy vegetables, 100–101
   timing of meals, 32
   vegetable choices, 55–57
   very lean meat, 58–59
   whole milk, 52
Meal-planning resources, 107
Meat choices
   high-fat meat, 62–63
   lean meat, 60–61
   meal planning, 57–63, 58*t*
   medium-fat meat, 61–62
   very lean meat, 58–59
Medical identification, 173–174
Medicines
   Acarbose (Precose), 128*t*
   Acetohexamide (Dymelor), 124*t*
   Actos (Pioglitazone), 127*t*
   Actos plus Met, 131*t*
   Albiglutide (Tanzeum), 133*t*, 134

Alfrezza, 136*t*
Alogliptin (Nesina), 129*t*
alpha-glucosidase inhibitors,
   128–129, 128*t*
Amaryl (Glimepiride), 124*t*
amylin mimetic, 134, 134*t*
Apidra, 136*t*, 142
Avandamet, 131*t*
Avandaryl, 131*t*
Avandia (Rosiglitazone), 127*t*
biguanides, 126–127, 126*t*
Bydureon (Exenatide extended
   release), 133*t*, 134
Byetta (Exenatide), 133*t*
Canagliflozin (Invokana), 130*t*
Chlorpropamide (Diabinese),
   124*t*, 125
Clear insulin, 142
Cloudy insulin, 142
combination medication,
   131*t*–132*t*, 133
Dapagliflozin (Farxiga), 130*t*
Diabeta (Micronase/Glyburide),
   124*t*
Diabinese (Chlorpropamide),
   124*t*, 125
double insulin, 142–144
DPP-4 inhibitor, 129, 129*t*
Dulaglutide (Trulicity), 133*t*, 134
Dymelor (Acetohexamide), 124*t*
Empagliflozin (Jardiance), 130*t*
Exenatide (Byetta), 133*t*
Farxiga (Dapagliflozin), 130*t*
Fortamet (Metformin), 126*t*
giving injection, 145–147
Glimepiride (Amaryl), 124*t*
Glipizide (Glucotrol), 124*t*, 125
Glipizide ER (Glucotrol XL), 124*t*
Glucophage (Metformin), 88,
   126–127, 126*t*
Glucophage XR (Metformin ER),
   126–127, 126*t*

Glucotrol (Glipizide), 124t, 125
Glucotrol XL (Glipizide ER), 124t
Glucovance, 131t
Glumetza (Metformin), 126t
Glyburide (Micronase/Diabeta), 124t
Glynase (Micronized Glyburide), 124t
Glyset (Miglitol), 128t
Glyxambi, 131t
Humalog, 135t, 142
Humalog Mix, 135t
Humulin N, 135t
Humulin R, 135t
important information, 137
incretin mimetic, 133–134, 133t
Inhaled Insulin, 136t
injection areas, 146–147
injection technique, 140–111
injection timings, 138
insulin, 140–142
insulin pen, 144
insulin pumps, 147–148
Invokamet, 132t
Invokana (Canagliflozin), 130t
Janumet, 131t
Janumet XR, 132t
Januvia (Sitagliptin), 129t
Jardiance (Empagliflozin), 130t
Jentadueto, 132t
Kazano, 132t
Kombliglyze XR, 131t
Lantus, 136t, 142
Levemir, 136t, 142
Lilly Insulin, 135t
Linagliptin (Tradjenta), 129t
Liraglutide (Victoza), 133t
meglitinides, 125–126, 125t
Metaglip, 131t
Metformin (Fortamet), 126t
Metformin (Glucophage), 88, 126–127, 126t

Metformin (Glumetza), 126t
Metformin ER (Glucophage XR), 126–127, 126t
Metformin liquid (Riomet), 126t
Micronase (Diabeta/Glyburide), 124t
Micronized Glyburide (Glynase), 124t
Miglitol (Glyset), 128t
Nesina (Alogliptin), 129t
Novolin 70/30, 136t
Novolin N, 136t
Novolog, 136t, 142
Novolog Mix, 136t
Novolog N, 136t
Novolog R, 136t
Novo Nordisk, 136t
Onglyza (Saxagliptin), 129t
oral, 196
Orinase (Tolbutamide), 124t
Oseni, 132t
Pioglitazone (Actos), 127t
Pramlinitide acetate, 134t
Prandimet, 131t
Precose (Acarbose), 128t
Regular, 142
Riomet (liquid Metformin), 126t
Rosiglitazone (Avandia), 127t
Sanofi, 136t
Saxagliptin (Onglyza), 129t
SGLT2 Inhibitor, 130, 130t
single insulin, 140–142
Sitagliptin (Januvia), 129t
storage, 138
Sulfa reactions, 124
sulfonylureas, 124–125, 124t
Symlin, 134t
Tanzeum (Albiglutide), 133t, 134
thiazolidinediones, 127–128, 127t
Tolazamide (Tolinase), 124t
Tolbutamide (Orinase), 124t
Tolinase (Tolazamide), 124t

Medicines (*continued*)
  Toujeo, 136*t*
  Tradjenta (Linagliptin), 129*t*
  Trulicity (Dulaglutide), 133*t*, 134
  Victoza (Liraglutide), 133*t*
  Xigduo XR, 132*t*
Medium-fat meat, 61–62
Meglitinides, 125–126, 125*t*
Metaglip, 131*t*
Metformin (Fortamet), 126*t*
Metformin (Glucophage), 88,
  126–127, 126*t*
Metformin (Glumetza), 126*t*
Metformin ER (Glucophage XR),
  126–127, 126*t*
Metformin liquid (Riomet), 126*t*
Microalbumin (urine test), 191
Micronase (Diabeta/Glyburide), 124*t*
Micronized Glyburide (Glynase), 124*t*
Miglitol (Glyset), 128*t*
Milk choices, 51*t*, 52
Monounsaturated fats, 41, 64

Nateglinide (Starlix), 125*t*
Nerve complications, 188–189
Nesina (Alogliptin), 129*t*
Neuropathy, 188
Nighttime hypoglycemia, 16
Non-insulin-dependent diabetes. *See*
  Type 2 diabetes
Novolin 70/30, 136*t*
Novolin N, 136*t*
Novolog, 136*t*, 142
Novolog Mix, 136*t*
Novolog N, 136*t*
Novolog R, 136*t*
Novo Nordisk, 136*t*
NutraSweet. *See* Aspartame
Nutrition Facts labels. *See* Food
  labels
Nuts, 106*t*

Obesity, 3, 196
Onglyza (Saxagliptin), 129*t*
Oral medicines, 196
  Acarbose (Precose), 128*t*
  Acetohexamide (Dymelor), 124*t*
  Actos (Pioglitazone), 127*t*
  Actos plus Met, 131*t*
  Albiglutide (Tanzeum), 133*t*, 134
  Alogliptin (Nesina), 129*t*
  alpha-glucosidase inhibitors,
    128–129, 128*t*
  Amaryl (Glimepiride), 124*t*
  amylin mimetic, 134, 134*t*
  Avandamet, 131*t*
  Avandaryl, 131*t*
  Avandia (Rosiglitazone), 127*t*
  biguanides, 126–127, 126*t*
  Bydureon (Exenatide extended
    release), 133*t*, 134
  Byetta (Exenatide), 133*t*
  Canagliflozin (Invokana), 130*t*
  causing blood sugar fluctuation,
    26*t*–27*t*
  Chlorpropamide (Diabinese),
    124*t*, 125
  combination medication,
    131*t*–132*t*, 133
  Dapagliflozin (Farxiga), 130*t*
  Diabeta (Micronase/Glyburide),
    124*t*
  Diabinese (Chlorpropamide),
    124*t*, 125
  DPP-4 inhibitor, 129, 129*t*
  Dulaglutide (Trulicity), 133*t*, 134
  Dymelor (Acetohexamide), 124*t*
  Empagliflozin (Jardiance), 130*t*
  Exenatide (Byetta), 133*t*
  Farxiga (Dapagliflozin), 130*t*
  Fortamet (Metformin), 126*t*
  Glimepiride (Amaryl), 124*t*
  Glipizide (Glucotrol), 124*t*, 125
  Glipizide ER (Glucotrol XL), 124*t*

Glucophage (Metformin), 88,
  126–127, 126t
Glucophage XR (Metformin ER),
  126–127, 126t
Glucotrol (Glipizide), 124t, 125
Glucotrol XL (Glipizide ER), 124t
Glucovance, 131t
Glumetza (Metformin), 126t
Glyburide (Micronase/Diabeta),
  124t
Glynase (Micronized Glyburide),
  124t
Glyset (Miglitol), 128t
Glyxambi, 131t
incretin mimetic, 133–134, 133t
Invokamet, 132t
Invokana (Canagliflozin), 130t
Janumet, 131t
Janumet XR, 132t
Januvia (Sitagliptin), 129t
Jardiance (Empagliflozin), 130t
Jentadueto, 132t
Kazano, 132t
Kombliglyze XR, 131t
Linagliptin (Tradjenta), 129t
Liraglutide (Victoza), 133t
meglitinides, 125–126, 125t
Metaglip, 131t
Metformin (Fortamet), 126t
Metformin (Glucophage), 88,
  126–127, 126t
Metformin (Glumetza), 126t
Metformin ER (Glucophage XR),
  126–127, 126t
Metformin liquid (Riomet), 126t
Micronase (Diabeta/Glyburide),
  124t
Micronized Glyburide (Glynase),
  124t
Miglitol (Glyset), 128t
Nateglinide (Starlix), 125t
Nesina (Alogliptin), 129t

Onglyza (Saxagliptin), 129t
Orinase (Tolbutamide), 124t
Oseni, 132t
Pioglitazone (Actos), 127t
Pramlinitide acetate, 134t
Prandimet, 131t
Prandin (Repaglinide), 125t
Precose (Acarbose), 128t
Repaglinide (Prandin), 125t
research about, 196
Riomet (liquid Metformin), 126t
Rosiglitazone (Avandia), 127t
Saxagliptin (Onglyza), 129t
SGLT2 Inhibitor, 130, 130t
Sitagliptin (Januvia), 129t
Starlix (Nateglinide), 125t
sulfonylureas, 124–125
Symlin, 134t
Tanzeum (Albiglutide), 133t, 134
thiazolidinediones, 127–128, 127t
Tolazamide (Tolinase), 124t
Tolbutamide (Orinase), 124t
Tolinase (Tolazamide), 124t
Tradjenta (Linagliptin), 129t
Trulicity (Dulaglutide), 133t, 134
Victoza (Liraglutide), 133t
Xigduo XR, 132t
Organizations, 199–201
Orinase (Tolbutamide), 124t
Oseni, 132t
Over-Eaters Anonymous, 196
Overweight, diet for, 31–32

Pancreas, 9, 9f, 195
Pasta, 44–45
Peas, 46
"Perfect meal," 9
Periodicals, 197, 200
Periodontal disease, 192
Personal hygiene. See Hygiene
Personalized meal plan, 78
Pioglitazone (Actos), 127t

Plate method, 69, 70f, 71t
Polyunsaturated fats, 41, 64
Post-prandial blood sugar test,
    149–150
Pramlinitide acetate, 134t
Prandimet, 131t
Prandin (Repaglinide), 125t
Precose (Acarbose), 128t
Pregnancy, 6, 196
Proteins, 7, 8–9, 40, 40f, 86
Pulse, measuring, 159–160

Quick Sticks, 20

Record keeping, blood-sugar tests
    and, 115
Reduced-fat milk, 52
Reduced-fat snacks, 32
Repaglinide (Prandin), 125t
Research, 195–196
Resources
    apps, 202–204
    books, 202, 204–206
    periodicals, 197, 200
    TV, 204
    Web resources, 201–202
Restaurants, eating at. See Dining
    out
Retinopathy, 189
Riomet (liquid Metformin), 126t
Risk factors for diabetes, 3, 6
Rosiglitazone (Avandia), 127t

Saccharin, 82
Salt. See Sodium
Sample meal plans
    Calories
    1500, 79t
    2000, 80t–81t
    high-fiber diet, 106t
    personalized meal plan, 78
    snacks guidelines, 77–81

Sanofi, 136t
Saturated fats, 41, 65, 99–101
Saxagliptin (Onglyza), 129t
Seasonings, 73–74
Seeds, 106t
Serving sizes, on food labels, 85 (see
    also Food portions)
SGLT2 Inhibitor, 130, 130t
Shopping tips, 89–90
Sick day plan, 165–168
Sickness, 26–28t, 28t. See also
    Diseases; specific illnesses
Sitagliptin (Januvia), 129t
Skin care, 170
Smoking, increasing complications
    and, 192
Snacks, 74–75
    guidelines for, 74–75, 76
    meal planning, 45, 82
    reduced-fat, 32
Sodium, 32, 86
Splenda. See Sucralose
Starches
    as fiber sources, 105t
    meal planning and, 43–47
    starch choices, 43–47
    starch foods prepared with fat,
        46–47
    starchy vegetables, 46
Starlix (Nateglinide), 125t
Stevia, 82
Stress
    exercise to reduce, 176
    hyperglycemia and, 175
    information sources, 177
    research about, 196
Stretching, 155
Sucralose, 82
Sugar. See Glucose
Sugar alcohols, 83
Sugar Twin. See Saccharin
Sulfa reactions, 124

Sulfonylureas, 124–125, 124*t*
Sunett. *See* Acesulfame-K
Support Groups, 196
Sweeteners, alternative. *See*
    Alternative sweeteners; *specific sweeteners*
Sweet'n Low. *See* Saccharin
Sweet One. *See* Acesulfame-K
Symlin, 134*t*
Symptoms
    of hyperglycemia, 13
    of hypoglycemia, 16–17, 17*f*
    ketone formation, 14, 14*f*
Syringes, insulin. *See* Insulin
    syringes

Tanzeum (Albiglutide), 133*t*, 134
Target ranges, 106*t*
    blood fat target, 100
    blood pressure, 193
    blood sugar, 28, 28*t*
    cholesterol, 193
    estimated Average Glucose, 193
    heart rate, 156–158, 158*t*
    Hemoglobin A1c, 193
Teeth and gum complications, 192
Tests. *See* Laboratory tests
Thiazolidinediones, 127–128, 127*t*
Tight blood sugar control, 111
Timing of meals, 32
Tolazamide (Tolinase), 124*t*
Tolbutamide (Orinase), 124*t*
Tolinase (Tolazamide), 124*t*
Total carbohydrate, on food labels, 86
Total fat, on food labels, 86
Toujeo, 136*t*
Tradjenta (Linagliptin), 129*t*

Trans fats, 30, 41, 100
Trans fatty acids. *See* Trans fats
Transportation Security
    Administration, 184
Traveling, 183–186
Triglycerides, 88
Trulicity (Dulaglutide), 133*t*, 134
Truvia. *See* Stevia
TSA. *See* Transportation Security
    Administration
TV programs, 204
Type 1 diabetes, 4, 10*t*
    diet for, 31 (*see also* Diet)
    research about, 195–196
Type 2 diabetes, 5, 10–11, 10*t*
    diet for, 31–32 (*see also* Diet)
    research about, 196

Urine ketone testing, 120–121

Vegetables
    as fiber sources, 104*t*–105*t*
    meal planning and, 55–57
Victoza (Liraglutide), 133*t*

Warm-up exercises, 155
Web resources
    for diabetics, 201–202
    fast food restaurant information, 98–99
Weight
    activity and, 32, 33
    healthy, 34–36
Weight reduction programs, 196
Weight Watchers, 196
Whole milk, meal planning, 52

Xigduo XR, 132*t*